Mothers
know best

What People are Saying about
Mothers Know Best

"*Mothers Know Best* has what every new mother needs: real advice from all kinds of folks, from moms to midwives to authors to nannies and more. Each entry is short and easy-to-read, so even the most exhausted new mother can get in a few valuable bits of advice between diaper changes. I wish I'd had a copy when I got home from the hospital with my newborn. That, and a full night's sleep, would have been just spectacular."

Jen Singer, author of *14 Hours 'Til Bedtime: A Stay-at-Home Mom's Life in 27 Funny Little Stories*

"New mothers are often inundated with advice. Sometimes the advice we get is just what we need to hear; all too often it's overwhelming. The beauty of this book is that it is a compilation of mothers' voices, in all their complexity. The suggestions in here, from real moms like you, are as differing as the mothers who wrote them, and yet they are all saying the same thing: I have been where you are, you will get through this, and you are not alone."

Andi Buchanan, author of *Mother Shock: Loving Every (Other) Minute of It*

"Full of warm and practical wisdom, this book nurtures mothers."

Pec Indman Ed.D., MFT, co-author of *Beyond the Blues, A Guide to Understanding and Treating Prenatal and Postpartum Depression*

"No one knows parenting like another parent. *Mothers Know Best* is like sitting down to a cup of coffee with your best girlfriend: you'll laugh, sigh, and ultimately (hopefully?) wind up motivated to get up and finish the dishes."

Sarah Smiley, syndicated columnist, author, and mother of two

"Reading *Mothers Know Best* is like sharing the laughter, tears, joys, and triumphs of motherhood with 1,001 of your best girlfriends. It is the ultimate support group for moms, right at your fingertips."

Deborah Shelton, author of *The Five Minute Parent: Fun & Fast Activities for You and Your Little Ones*

Real Moms Share
1001 Tips on Pregnancy,
Birth and the First Year

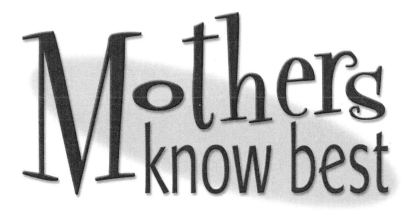

Edited by Connie Correia Fisher and Joanne Correia

Foreword by Dr. Jennifer L. Howse

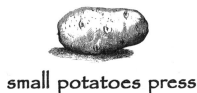

small potatoes press

ISBN: 0-9661200-6-X
Library of Congress Control Number: 2004099879

Fisher, Connie Correia.
  Mother knows best : real moms share 1001 tips on pregnancy, birth and the first
year / Connie Correia Fisher, Joanne Correia. - Collingswood, NJ : Small
Potatoes Press, 2005.
  348 p. ; 24 cm.
  ISBN 0-9661200-6-X
  1. Pregnancy — Popular works. 2. Childbirth. 3. Infants – Care. 4. Motherhood.
I. Correia, Joanne. II. Title.
RG525 F533 2005
618.24

Printed in the United States

10 9 8 7 6 5 4 3 2 1

Small Potatoes Press
401 Collings Avenue
Collingswood, NJ 08108
856-869-5207
www.smallpotatoespress.com

Dedication

For wise mothers everywhere, especially these amazing moms...
Christine, Cindy, Dawn, Debbie, Kathi, Kelly,
Meredith, Robyn, and Stacy...
and the moms we miss...Sylvia, Marie, Anne, and Ruth

Table of

Pregnancy

Birth

Baby's First Year

Contents

Your First Year

Special Deliveries

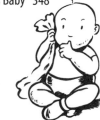

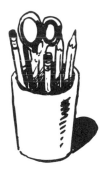

Introduction

When I became pregnant, the thing I needed more than ice cream and a better bra was advice. I had lots of books but no time to read them. I had an OB who had no time to talk. Luckily, I had friends and relatives with babies and even some who were pregnant at the same time I was. And I had my mom, the original super hero of mothers. From the time I found out I was pregnant until this morning, I must have called my mother four times a day. Not everyone is so fortunate to have such a support staff, yet there were still days I really needed to know that other moms were afraid of the snot-sucking nose bulb and more than a little concerned that their hair was falling out in clumps.

Now that I've been a mom for a few years, it's funny to me that newbie moms ask ME for advice. Me? Surely they know that I am only winging this mommy thing. What I've learned from creating *Mothers Know Best* is that we all are. We're all winging it and learning from our triumphs and mistakes; all sharing, all scared and tired, joyful, uncertain and proud — sometimes all at the same time. And it really helps to be able to share these feelings with someone who is or was in the same place —someone who has pushed the stroller around the proverbial block and tells it like it is with compassion, understanding, and often, humor.

The 500 moms who contributed tips to *Mothers Know Best* do just that. Their tips are geared to help pregnant and new moms adjust and enjoy this amazing and sometimes stressful time and not to lecture or judge. And with advice from so many moms, one thing is clear: there is no ONE WAY to do anything, and every mom has times of doubt, anxiety, and, ultimately, success. Each pregnancy, birth, and baby is extraordinary, personal, and life-changing.

Something else that is life-changing is the March of Dimes. Since the mid-1990s, I have done some fund-raising here or there for the March of Dimes, but the fight became much more personal when my son was born 12 weeks premature in 2001. A therapy—which March of Dimes helped to fund and perfect— saved his life. Now I am much more aware of the incredible work they do and am so pleased that 25 cents from the sale of each copy of *Mothers Know Best* will go directly to their fight against premature birth and birth defects.

I hope that *Mothers Know Best* gives you hope, courage, and confidence in your decisions. After all, who knows more about the highs and lows, ins and outs of surviving and enjoying pregnancy, birth, and a child's first year than a mom?

Connie Correia Fisher
(Joanne's daughter and co-editor of *Mothers Know Best*)

Doing this book with my daughter Connie has opened my eyes as to how times have changed since I gave birth to her 36 years ago. Not only times but technology and terms are different. Today's moms are out and about much sooner after delivery. (I was instructed to stay in for three weeks and to use stairs only on a limited basis.) Baby "super markets" stock EVERYTHING you could possibly need or want. NICU's are state of the art; ultrasounds have become routine, revealing much, including the sex of the baby. (My four were all surprises!) Words like "doula" and "white noise" are now part of my vocabulary; "sling" has taken on a new meaning (always thought it was something to use when you broke your arm). Entire families can now witness the birth thanks to birth centers, a far cry from curtained labor rooms and white tiled no-dads-allowed delivery rooms. And if the family can't be present, all the excitement can be captured on a digital camera and uploaded to a customized Web site.

But fortunately, some things haven't changed…important things like "love your babies," "trust your instincts," and above all, "enjoy the moments." Trust me: the time DOES go by much too quickly. Before you know it, your babies are having babies of their own.

Joanne Correia
(Connie's mom and co-editor of *Mothers Know Best*)

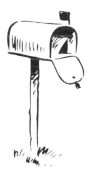

Foreword

"Mothers are the most instinctive philosophers," wrote Harriet Beecher Stowe. The March of Dimes, a nonprofit health agency dedicated to improving the health of America's mothers and babies, applauds the wisdom of moms throughout our country.

President Franklin D. Roosevelt established the March of Dimes in 1938 to address the worsening epidemics of the paralyzing disease polio that were then sweeping the nation. He created a partnership of volunteer moms and dads and researchers so effective that, within 17 years, the Salk polio vaccine had been developed, and this terrible disease was halted in the U.S.

Today the March of Dimes, in partnership with the American Academy of Pediatrics, recommends that all babies receive vaccinations that protect them from a dozen very serious diseases such as measles, mumps and rubella. For more information, including the complete vaccination schedule, visit our Web site at www.marchofdimes.com.

Fighting Premature Birth

Prematurity is now the most serious, common, and costly problem affecting newborns in America. Each year, more than 470,000 babies (1 in 8) are born too soon, some so small they can fit in the palm of a hand. Many of these babies must fight just to survive; others face lifelong health problems. No one knows the causes of nearly half of all premature births, and no one is working harder than the March of Dimes to find out. To learn more about the risks factors for prematurity, and the warning signs and symptoms of preterm labor, visit the March of Dimes Prematurity Campaign Web site at www.marchofdimes.com/prematurity.

Education

The March of Dimes Pregnancy & Newborn Health Education Center^{SM} on the Web features information on a wide variety of topics related to your healthy pregnancy, including getting ready for parenthood, prenatal testing, good nutrition during pregnancy, birth defects and genetics, and caring for your baby after birth. The topic of loss is addressed with an array of sensitive bereavement materials. In addition, the Center is staffed by Health Information Specialists who can answer your questions by e-mail at askus@marchofdimes.com

Newborn Screening

In 2000 the March of Dimes led the way in proposing a national standard for newborn screening with a minimum core list of certain disorders for which every state should provide testing for every baby. Today the March of Dimes recommends that every baby receive testing at birth for about 30 life-threatening or disabling conditions for which immediate treatment is needed. Learn more about these disorders and why your baby needs newborn screening on the March of Dimes Web site at www.marchofdimes/nbs.

With the help and support of the American people and companies like Small Potatoes Press, the March of Dimes has helped protect the lives and the health of millions of moms and babies over the past 65 years. We won't stop until we reach the day when every baby has the chance to be born healthy.

Regards,
Dr. Jennifer L. Howse
President, March of Dimes

Pregnancy

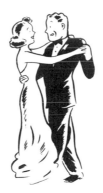

Ready for Baby?

It is best to conceive when you are only 75% sure. There's never the absolute perfect time: you always want to lose that extra five pounds, gain a bigger savings account, or reorganize the house. Seventy-five percent means your heart and your head are aligned. That's as good as it gets!

**Wendy, counselor and mother of Katie, age 14 months, and Baby #2 on the way
New Jersey**

Pregnancy and childbirth are major life events, but the hardest part comes after delivery. Raising children to be successful adults requires extreme amounts of parental time, energy, and attention for the next twenty years or so. I see too many children these days who obviously are not getting the parenting they need. This is evident in the neighborhoods, shopping malls, schools, and police reports. Readers of this book need to consider why they want to become parents and if they are up to the challenge.

**Jane, PFLAG
Anchorage**

Naprotechnology is a new reproductive science that works with the woman's cycle. Thank God for this program. It brought us a healthy Naprotechnology baby boy, naturally. www.fertilitycare.org.

**Leslie, mother of Connor William, age 16 months
Ontario, Canada**

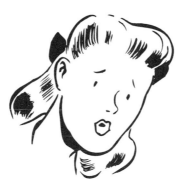

Emotions

Contrary to popular mythology, pregnancy is not always a happy, glowing experience! Approximately 15 to 20 percent of pregnant women experience depression. Of these, about 15 percent are so severely depressed that they attempt suicide. When symptoms of depression or other mood disorders cause limitations in the client's ability to function on a day-to-day basis, intervention is necessary.
This may include traditional (counseling and medication) or nontraditional (such as Yoga or acupressure) modalities, or any combination thereof. The goal is to use whatever the individual woman needs in order to feel like herself again.

Shoshana S. Bennett, Ph.D., mother of Elana and Aaron and Pec Indman, Ed.D., MFT, mother of Megan and Emily: co-authors of *Beyond the Blues, A Guide to Understanding and Treating Prenatal and Postpartum Depression*
California

Trust your body and do not fear the unknown. Educate yourself as much as you can. Do not be afraid to ask your doctor or midwife questions. Ask and keep asking to ensure the same answer. Surround yourself with like-minded people, and, most of all, hire a labor doula to help you and your partner through the beautiful journey into childbirth.

**Rosemarie, labor support doula and mother of
John, age 11, and Nicholas, age 8
New Jersey**

Not every pregnancy is expected, and even those that are planned may create mixed emotions once the hormone roller coaster gets set into motion. The best thing that helped me to start bonding with my tiny, unborn baby was to go out and buy something for the little one. It started with a pair of little booties and moved on to shoes, books, and clothes. It doesn't have to be expensive, but it really helps to have something concrete that "belongs" to baby for you to hold and look at.

It's a nice time to indulge in fun things for baby, because once the reality of diapers, wipes, food, and so much more sets in, it may be much harder to buy those adorable but so unpractical little things.

**Kate, counselor and mother of Isabella, age 17 months
New Jersey**

I had a mantra I kept saying to myself during my first pregnancy and unmedicated delivery: "I trust the wisdom of my body and the instincts of my baby." I found it to be soothing and reassuring. I have been using it during this pregnancy as well. I find it reconnects me to the birthing legacies of centuries of mothers who've gone before.

**Katherine, S-LP and mother of
Elahna Claire, age 31 months, and new addition due early October 2004
Ontario, Canada**

There's a lot I know for sure and a lot more that I will learn. I know that motherhood is the scariest, most challenging, most rewarding, and most important job that you will ever have. I know that it makes you feel vulnerable yet incredibly strong at the same time. The instinct to protect your child is in every fiber of your being, and it comes out with a vengeance once you become a mother. God has blessed me with two beautiful girls. My girls are 3 years old and 2½ months old. I am in awe of them daily. I am forever changed by becoming a mother. I have discovered that the gifts I get from this journey, good and challenging, are shaping me as a person and have provided the fulfillment that I had been searching for prior to becoming pregnant with my first daughter. I still have so much to learn. Everyone's experience is different. Embrace the journey, moms-to-be. It's the ride of your life. The irony of it all is that you find out that the things your parents said to you when you were growing up ARE TRUE, and you will find yourself smiling when you sound just like them.

**Lea, courtesy of The Center for Conscious Parenting, www.cfcp.info,
mother of two little gems ages 3 and 2½ months
Oregon**

Shield family and friends from raging pregnancy hormones by recording your thoughts, rants, and tirades in a journal. You will feel better, and people won't be afraid to be around you.

Deborah Shelton, author of *The Five Minute Parent: Fun & Fast Activities for You and Your Little Ones* and mother of Kizer, age 6

Start loving your baby/child from conception. Communicate with your baby: tell him/her about yourself, family, friends, what you are feeling during the pregnancy. Maintain loving relationships with others.

**Cecile Peterkin, president of Cosmic Coaching Centre, publisher of *Recipe for Success* a monthly e-zine, and involved aunt of nephew Josh, age 15, and niece Jordash, age 13
Toronto, Canada**

The most important tip I can think of is TIME: time to enjoy every aspect of your pregnancy; all of the feelings of this unknown soul growing inside of you. Every sense, every emotion is to be cherished. Once your little bundle of joy has emerged, treasure every moment of new growth and discovery, for every moment is a precious gift not to be taken for granted or cast aside. Relax — do not stress. Just sit back and hold this special gift in your arms and thank your God for blessing you with this creation. The greatest gift we can give our children is our time, our full attention, and our unconditional love.

**Heidi, business owner and mother of Caitlyn Jean, age 14 months
Idaho**

Stay as peaceful and positive as you can throughout your pregnancy. How we moms respond is how our little ones' personalities are formed.

**Angela, virtual secretary and mother of
Michael, age 15, Caldonia, age 7, and Kathryn, age 12 months
Illinois**

I thought the more I read, the better prepared I would be. This is true to an extent. But sometimes, too much knowledge can make you more terrified than you already are. Read enough to educate yourself about where you are. Don't start to read about the delivery while in your first few months: it can be too much. Pace yourself on a need-to-know basis.

**Christine, full-time diva and mother of Julia, age 2½, and Olivia, age 6 months
New Jersey**

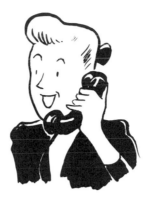

Telling Everyone

When we were expecting our fourth baby, we really wanted to do something different. Our youngest at the time was 2½ years old. So, we took an old T-shirt and with permanent black ink wrote on the front "I'm going to be a big sister!" And then we just let her walk into the living room where all my family was sitting. It didn't take long for my youngest brother, James (19 at the time), to notice and leap up with an exclamation of "You're pregnant? Alright!" The faces of everyone else were priceless as they tried to clue in to what was going on!

Nicole, doula and mother of Alanna, age 8, Braden, age 6,
Danielle, age 3, and Ethan, age 2 months
Canada

A memorable way to announce your pregnancy is to put your baby's first ultrasound in an ultrasound picture frame (like the Images by Ellyn Sonogram Keepsake Frames), wrap it up, and give it to grandma and grandpa. It'll tell them your good news AND be a memorable keepsake.

Sherry Bonelli, www.PregnancyStore.com, and mother of
Connor, age 6, and twins Sidney and Kiley, age 2
Illinois

When my husband and I decided to start trying to have our first child, I had planned out in my mind how I would tell him of the blessed event. I figured I would find out by myself and then plan a romantic dinner — candles, lobster…the whole thing. Then, I planned to give him a card and a gift congratulating him on becoming a father. (You know, one of those cards that speak to the expectant father?) He would look confused for a second and look at me over the candle light and say, "You are pregnant?" and I would exclaim, "Yes!" Then we would hug and revel in the moment, the moment that would change our lives forever. Well, you know what they say about best laid plans. That was the vision; now here is what really happened. It was early one Sunday morning in September. I felt changes happening to my body. I hadn't missed my period yet because it was not due for another five days. I bought pregnancy tests the day before. I just had, you know, that feeling. So I woke up around 6:30 am, and I decided to perform the test. I could not wait any longer. I read the directions and performed the test. The first line showed up immediately; then faintly I noticed a second line (one, not pregnant; two, pregnant). I read the directions again. "Okay, I think there are two lines." I needed confirmation of this. Was my mind playing tricks on me, or were there really two lines? All I could think about was, "I think I am pregnant, I think I am pregnant. I need someone to make sure what I am seeing is really there." (The plans for the wonderful romantic dinner went right out the window.) My husband was the only other person that could confirm my findings at this time – it would have to be him. I ran out into the bedroom around to his side of the bed and started shaking him violently, shouting "Are there two lines, are there two lines?" as I stuck this urine-soaked stick in his face. He looked at me like I had gone off the deep end and said, "Yes." That's how my husband found out I was pregnant with Sophia.

(P.S. After he said, "Yes," he then asked, "Is there pee on that thing? Get that out of my face! Yuck." Very romantic, indeed.)

Dawn, RN, and mother of Sophia, age 3, and Analiese, age 1
New Jersey

If your husband or partner isn't there when you take the pregnancy test, creatively clue him into the big news, even if it's just so you have a good story to tell. You can "accidentally" leave the pregnancy test out for him to find, rent him a few baby-related movies, give him a card, or write him a love note. Whichever way you decide to tell him, he will be overjoyed and excited to start this new phase of his life with you.

Kristen, mother of Elise, age 1
North Dakota

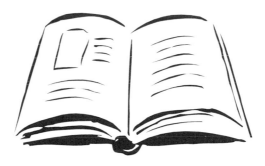

Must Reads & Resources

The book *Happy Baby, Healthy Sleep Habits* by Dr. Marc Weissbluth is a must have.

Elisa, management consultant and mother of Quinn, age 17 months
Colorado

The Womanly Art of Breastfeeding is the one book you need to learn how and why to breastfeed. It is also the source of wisdom from breastfeeding mothers for nearly 50 years. Read it before the baby arrives and you'll turn back to it again and again.

Stephanie, mother of Kate, age 8, and Ben, age 6
Maryland

Read *The Plug-In Drug* by Marie Win and find out how much fun being face-to-face is without a television in your baby's life!

Sarah, civil engineer and mother of a little boy, age 2½
New York

These Web sites are great sites for moms: www.breastfeeding.com, www.mothering.com, and www.gentlemothering.com.

Heather, registered nurse
South Carolina

Have these on hand so that you can reference them when you are trying to figure out what to do next, whether you and your baby are normal, the anticipations for the next joys and challenges. The first two espouse the Eat-Wake-Sleep cycle. I needed both of them, however, to really learn how to, when to, and when not to do the things that made my baby a good eater and sleeper. FYI: They do not support the family bed concept.

Babywise by Gary Ezzo and Robert Bucknam: Not especially well-written, but a real how-to primer for you to teach baby good eating and sleeping habits — really your only job in the early months besides loving and kissing and hugging baby. I didn't adopt the part about letting the baby cry to sleep because I also read....

Secrets of the Baby Whisperer by Tracy Hogg: This book is more comprehensive, better written, and more gentle than *Babywise*. (It was also a better match to my own style.) She also has good tips about breast-feeding.

The Happiest Baby on the Block: Developed by a California doctor, it teaches you four key ways to stop a baby from crying, and it teaches you why they cry. It really works! (There is a video and a book, although I think his techniques must be seen on video to really understand them.)

Dr. Spocks's Baby and Child Care: A good all-around health, behavior, and development reference, although it doesn't seem to know about Eat-Wake-Sleep, so don't look to it for eating/sleeping issues.

Sleeping Through the Night: At 4 to 6 weeks, this is a good reference to read to get ready for baby to start working toward sleeping through the night. While *Baby Whisperer* drove the routine, this book provides more alternatives and choices for you to consider.

The contributing moms of "The List,"
a growing list of new mom tips passed from friend to friend
New Jersey, Maryland, and Delaware

The internet is a great resource for baby information. Whenever I have questions or concerns, I'll do research (so easy to do online) so that I can make up my own mind or have some thoughts to share with the pediatrician. Always go with what you feel is best (no matter what your family or friends say) and stay INFORMED!

Kristi, technical support and mother of Ethan, age 5 months
Washington

Anything by Penny Simkin!

Ilana Stein, doula trainer and mentor and childbirth educator
New York

The internet is a great tool for new mothers. However, for those who are seeking advice or help, it can be a scary and confusing place filled with conflicting information that attempts to answer questions that only you and your baby (through trial and error) will get the true answers to.

Jennifer, Web designer and mother of Scarlett, age 4 months
New Jersey

The best book I have ever seen on pregnancy is a book called *Birth* by Rachel Broncher. I lent it to everyone I knew. She's Australian, from Melbourne, and it is unlike the traditional pregnancy books. If you are interested in breathing techniques and meditation, etc., you will love it. It's very calming and soothing, has some great exercises, and great photographs. Different mothers talk about their labor and birth experiences, which I found very interesting. Some were first time mums; others were on their third, fourth, fifth, etc., child. Many confirmed how much better their births were using Rachel's techniques compared to previous births. I always found breathing better during labor than anything else, and I had four very different labors. I thought it was a wonderful book and read it throughout each of my pregnancies.

Nanette, teacher and mother of
Kara, age 9, Zoe, age 7, Jed, age 6, and Dom, age 2
London, United Kingdom

The Thinking Woman's Guide to a Better Birth by Henci Goer.

Colleen Holland, doctor of chiropractic and mother of Amelia, age 9 months
Colorado

Don't consider anything you read in any book to be the golden rule. The author of that or any book was not writing with your baby in mind. Go with your instinct – it's usually correct.

Susan, analyst and mother of Peter Kent, age 3
Pennsylvania

Use your community telephone book for many unknown resources for mom and baby.

Dolores, R.N., Lamaze (LCCE), doula, and mother of Jonathon and Megan
New York

Happiest Baby on the Block gave me the information and tips I needed to calm baby and survive the fourth trimester! Read before baby arrives and you'll enjoy baby's first few months of life!

Amy Tardio, therapist, counselor, and mother of John, age 1
Illinois

Listen to your baby's needs and tune into your own instincts. The very best read is *The Womanly Art of Breastfeeding* published by La Leche League. Joining this organization to support women is certainly a very smart thing to do.

Silke, mother of Melanie, age 8, and Hannah, age 6
Bramley, Great Britain

Here's some of the best sources of information on children's well-being.

Children's Defense Fund (www.childrensdefense.org), working since 1973 under the leadership of Marian Wright Edelman, has been advocating for all children in the US. It's the best place to find information about children's well-being in the US.

UNICEF (www.unicef.org): As a part of the United Nations, UNICEF advocates for children in 158 countries and territories around the world. We all know UNICEF, but it's a site you have to visit to understand UNICEF's amazing impact. You name it, you'll find it here.

Mothers Acting Up (www.mothersactingup.org) is a movement to summon the gigantic political strength of mothers and others to ensure the health, education, and safety of every child, not just a privileged few. Find easy monthly actions to do and the education around these issues to know why they are so important.

Free the Children (www.freethechildren.org) was started by a 12-year-old boy in 1995 to free children from slavery, poverty, and exploitation. As an international network of children helping children on all levels, the organization is also freeing children and young people from the idea that they are powerless to bring about positive social change and to improve the lives of their peers.

Every Child Matters (www.everychildmatters.org) promotes the adoption of smart policies for children and families by making children's needs a national political priority. Visit their Web site for a free "I'm voting for Kids" bumper sticker!

Kidsactingup.org (www.kidsactingup.org): Join MAU kids in acting up.

Beth Osnes, co-founder of Mothers Acting Up, part-time instructor of theatre at University of Colorado, and mother of Peter, age 11, Melisande, age 9, and Lerato, age 1, just adopted from South Africa!
Colorado

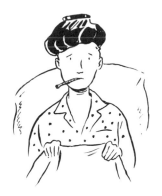

Sick and Tired

When you begin to feel nauseous, take a raw lemon and cut it in half. Squeeze and slowly drink the juice directly from the lemon. I tried just about everything else, and this really did take the edge off the nausea.

Kathi, mother of Matthew, age 6, Allison, age 4, and Miranda, age 6 months
Alabama

Use seabands. They make you look like a fool, but they worked WONDERS for me.

Jill, accountant/HR and mother of Sara, age 8, and Ethan, age 1
Canada

Believe it or not, a glass of soy milk does a wonderful job of preventing and curing this nasty problem. Rather than end the pregnancy to save her life, my sister agreed to drink a glassful every two hours, and her severe nausea came to an end. I found it helps mild nausea, too.

Kathleen, business executive, homeschool advocate, and mother of
John, age 42, Jean, age 39, Jim, age 37, Joe, age 29, Jesse, age 25,
plus thirteen grandkids – all homeschooled!
Chile

Hopefully it will miss you. But if it doesn't, do whatever your body tells you. Throw out rules about fruit and veggies if they make you sick, and you can only eat tacos. Make sure to eat something at least every three hours. Keep crackers by your bed when you wake up, and keep some ginger ale in the fridge.

Tracy, director of Christian education and mother of
Hannah, age 2, and Christian, age 4 months
Pennsylvania

Quick care for headache, mild cramping, or constipation: drink three glasses of water in quick succession. Drink three glasses in a half an hour. This works much of the time as many discomforts are caused by dehydration. A bath is also good.

Andrea, doula and mother of Christina, age 8
Canada

Always keep something in your stomach. Focus on proteins. If you eat crackers, have protein with it. Almonds, cashews, sunflower seeds…always keep something in your pocket. Almonds are great: you can suck on them or chew them slowly if you need to. However, ration them as you shouldn't eat too many in a day – about half a cup. Also, sipping pure ginger tea works great.

Andrea, doula and mother of Christina, age 8
Canada

A quick and healthy way to get rid of heartburn, as yucky as it sounds, is apple cider vinegar. The best kind to get (for health benefit as well as taste) is the unfiltered kind from the health food store, but distilled will work in a pinch. Place 1 teaspoon to 1 tablespoon of the apple cider vinegar in a couple ounces of water. You may add a little honey, if you wish. Mix it and drink it down. If you are using distilled, it may burn a little for a second, but the heartburn will then be gone.

Marisa, mother of Elijah, age 2½, and Marin, age 9 months
California

Ginger snaps or ginger ale work wonders. Wintergreen lifesavers also help.

Carlene, teacher and mother of Kate, age 7, and Jack, age 1

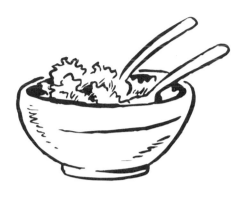

Eating for Two

Avoid overeating while pregnant. Eat smaller meals more frequently and drink lots of water. When you feel full, stop immediately! Eat small desserts once a week to decrease sugar cravings.

Jeanine B. Downie, M.D., dermatologist and mother of Jude, age 1½
New Jersey

The best advice I received for eating while pregnant was to try to make sure that everything I ate had some nutritional value. When deciding what to eat for a snack, I would keep that in mind and have a cup of yogurt and an apple rather than a donut or a bagel. When you do that, you can eat when you're hungry, feel good about providing your baby with the nutrients she needs, and not worry about gaining too much weight. That said, from time to time, you do have to make exceptions for your own sanity and happiness. I mean, really, ice cream has calcium, and chocolate does have some nutritional value. (I even read in an article that babies whose moms ate chocolate were happier!)

Cathy, mother of Maggie, age 5 weeks
Ohio

My tip is to eat as healthy as possible! (I tried to eat healthy, but nothing ever stayed in.) Eating healthy is the best thing you can do for yourself and your growing baby.

Tracy, stay-at-home mother of Sydney, age 26 months
California

I was extremely careful with my diet. I usually abstained from "unnecessary calories." I drank plenty of water and milk, but not after 5:30 pm. That way I usually got a good and uninterrupted night's sleep. I always broiled my meat and never used high sodium seasonings. For many women, low sodium foods help reduce swelling. Good nutrition is important through life. There are many good books on the subject, but I recommend *Nutrition Almanac* (now in its fourth printing). *Nutrition Almanac* will help you and your baby stay healthy for many, many years!

Judy Roy, inventor of Judy's Bottle Holder and mother of
Debra, age 24, and Katherine, age 20
Virginia

Don't let yourself "go" when you're pregnant and say, "I can eat like I always wanted to because I'm pregnant." When the pregnancy is over, then you're just fat.

Leigh Donadieu, publisher of *Cuizine* magazine and mother of
Mitchell, age 4, and Ruth, age 2
New Jersey

This was the most difficult part of pregnancy – always being hungry. Have plenty of good snacks — nuts, fruit, crackers, protein bars, shakes — for when you have not cooked and for in between meals. You need to eat more than you think.

Diane Hynes, shiatsu/craniosacral practitioner and mother of
Taegan, age 28 months
New Jersey

Take tons of calcium supplements to keep the "Charlie horses" away. Don't forget to flex your foot rather than point it when you to get one to help avoid the pain that follows.

Heidi, teacher and mother of Elisabeth, age 4, and Lauren, age 2
California

Remember…you ARE eating for two, but it's one adult and one baby.

Jennifer, certified childbirth educator and mother of
Amanda, age 5½, and Abby, age 2½
Georgia

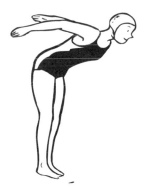

Exercise

Exercising as long as possible really helped with my delivery, mostly in the stamina department. And those Breathe Right™ strips helped a TON when I was completely congested (the entire pregnancy).

Alicia, mother of William, age 1
New Jersey

It was my experience that being able to maintain a moderate exercise program during my pregnancy helped my energy levels and helped with the endurance sometimes required during labor. This same practice was also key in returning me to my prepregnancy body after delivery.

Laurie Bagley, owner of Fit Maternity & Beyond and mom to Avriel, age 7
California

Even if you have never taken yoga before becoming pregnant, I highly recommend taking prenatal yoga classes and then continue doing yoga all the way up to the day you deliver. Doing prenatal yoga helps strengthen your pelvic floor while preparing you mentally for delivery. Controlled conscious breathing (pranayama) is an integral component of yoga that you will definitely use in the birthing room.

Andrea, desktop support specialist and mother of
Leah Athena, age 1 month
New Jersey

When I was pregnant with my second child, unhappy with the extra pounds I was still carrying from my first pregnancy, I took a class offered through my hospital called "Fit for Delivery." The class was run by a physical therapist who spent the first hour of class discussing topics such as nutrition and body mechanics and comfort techniques such as proper bending, lifting, and relaxation breathing. Afterward, we were put through the paces of a safe 45-minute exercise session. I was shocked at how much I learned. My OB was fantastic, but outside of telling me how much weight I'd gained and what my blood pressure was, he wasn't really giving me a lot of information about my changing body. A fitness class such as the one I took, designed specifically for pregnant women, was invaluable. I felt better, was less exhausted, and lost my "baby fat" much quicker the second time around.

**Judy Davids, guitarist for the all-mom rock band The Mydols and mother of
Dylan, age 11, and William, age 9
Michigan**

When I was pregnant, especially my first trimester, I found that exercise helped alleviate my queasiness! Of course, I recommend checking with your doctor before starting an exercise program if you haven't exercised pre-pregnancy.

**Kelly, fitness specialist and mother of Isabella, age 10 months
Texas**

I have taught prenatal and postnatal yoga for 10 years. It is a foundational practice for mothers and their babies. It strengthens the physical body, stabilizes the mental body, and quiets and focuses the mind – thus allowing the brain to be calm.

**Shosha, yoga instructor and mother of
Cecilia, age 23, and Clara Inez, age 19
California**

Remember that moms set the example for their families in terms of healthy eating and physical activity. Be a great role model for your family by making exercise a part of every day, even before you actually become a mom! Start your exercise routine during pregnancy, then continue it throughout your life. You will be setting an awesome example!

**Lisa Stone, pre/postnatal fitness specialist and mother of
Emma, age 15½, Savannah, age 13, and Morgan, age 8
Georgia**

Many women want to make lifestyle changes when they find out they are pregnant and are more open to experiencing new forms of exercise and spiritual growth. Yoga is an excellent form of exercise that provides perfect preparation for childbirth. Most women can safely begin a yoga practice at any point in their pregnancy, but they will want to find a teacher who is knowledgeable about the issues of pregnancy. Search the internet for prenatal yoga classes in your area and don't be afraid to call the teacher and ask questions.

Ann, Lamaze certified birth educator, certified prenatal yoga teacher, and mother of Ben, age 12, and Stephen, age 10
Maryland

My pregnancies and childbirths were easy and enjoyable. I attribute this BLESSING partly to genetics and partly to my healthy lifestyle. I always exercised and didn't quit just because I was expecting. I did, however, change my routine and hired a trainer to show me "pregnancy safe" exercises. My favorite exercise was swimming. It helps you relax. It makes the baby exercise also, and this helps baby and you sleep. Exercising helps your body adjust to the numerous changes it is undergoing. And it helps you to feel good about them.

Judy Roy, inventor of Judy's Bottle Holder and mother of Debra, age 24, and Katherine, age 20
Virginia

It is very important that you maintain some sort of exercise. You will feel much better afterwards.

Carla, paralegal and mother of Ashley, age 10
Missouri

Fresh air may help you avoid headaches. I had frequent headaches with my first two pregnancies. After getting the second one in my third pregnancy, I realized I hadn't been outside for two days. I took a walk every single day after that and never had another headache.

Susan Gmeiner, president of Maya Wrap and mother of Arj, age 14, Michael, age 12, and Karl, age 4
North Carolina

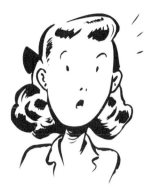

Embarrassments

My husband believes all pregnant women share a "fart conspiracy" where we pass intestinal gas at will, justifying our flatulence by our pregnant status. I have tried to dissuade his point of view, but no matter. As a mother-to-be, you will find yourself implicated in the conspiracy. I am not sure there is much you can do about it, other than, perhaps, blame it on Fido.

Celeste Palermo, freelance writer and mother of Peyton, age 6, and Morgan, age 1
Colorado

A lot of women get hemorrhoids during pregnancy or after birth. I was really embarrassed that I had a hemorrhoid until the nurse told me that she got one after her second child, and a lot of women get them when they have children. Don't stress about it. (Most women are too embarrassed to talk about this problem.) I guess it is just a part of becoming a mom.

Lori, advertising project manager and mother of Lincoln, age 18 months

Soak a makeup pad with witch hazel and wear it inside a pair of thong underwear around the house or at bedtime to relieve hemorrhoids.

Sarah, doula, ECE, and mother
Canada

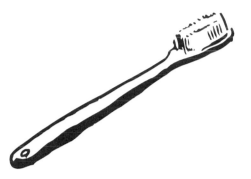

— Taking Care of Yourself —

Fifty to seventy-five percent of pregnant women get gingivitis; a bacterial infection characterized by red, tender, puffy, and often bleeding gums. Since a bacterial infection has the potential to trigger premature delivery, it is very important to make sure that a mother-to-be takes care of her oral health even before she conceives. Prenatal dental visits are vitally important in supporting whole body health. Brushing with an effective antibacterial toothpaste (one with baking soda and peroxide, such as Arm and Hammer), flossing daily, and using a dental irrigator (such as a Water-pik) with a bacteria fighting mouthwash is important for maintaining good oral health.

Sheila Wolf, registered dental hygienist, author of
Pregnancy and Oral Health: The Critical Connection Between Your Mouth and Your Baby,
and mother of Alan, age 31
California

Postpartum depression can begin during pregnancy and/or immediately after birth or any time during the first year after birth. For more information, visit www.ppdsupport.org and www.postpartum.net.

Helena Bradford, Chm., The Ruth Craven Foundation
for Postpartum Depression Awareness
South Carolina

Protect your baby and pamper yourself during pregnancy! Hire a midwife who will treat you like a healthy mom and get a doula who can support your birth goals.

Kelley, childbirth educator and mother of Simon, age 2
Massachusetts

Essential oils and flower essences such as Bach Flower Essences can correct emotional imbalances: negative emotions are replaced with positive. The following scents and Essences can be especially helpful during pregnancy.

Elm: This Essence helps us when we feel that things are too overwhelming. Being pregnant can be overwhelming: our body is growing and changing; moreover, we have to handle our job, family responsibilities, maybe other children. We are overwhelmed by responsibilities. Elm helps us restore our normal capable personality and helps us take time to look after our own needs.

Mustard: This Essence helps us when we for no apparent reason get depressed. Suddenly the depression comes and goes for no known reason. We are supposed to be happy and excited, but we experience a sudden depression that overcasts everything and destroys our normal cheerfulness. Mustard restores our inner stability and peace of mind and brings joy to our life.

Crab Apple: This helps us when we get to the point where we have grown out of our clothes, and we are standing in front of the mirror feeling like an elephant. No matter how beautiful our husband tells us that we look, we feel huge. Crab Apple helps us accept that we are carrying a baby in our belly. We are supposed to be huge. We will be able to look in the mirror and see a pregnant woman, not an elephant.

Olive: This Essence helps us when we feel utterly exhausted. Pregnancy can be terribly exhausting for our body, and we need extra sleep. Olive helps us restore our strength and vitality when all our energy has run out. If you are very tired, please see a doctor to check for nutritional or physical reasons as well.

Bettina Rasmussen, co-owner of PlatyPaws Soft Soles Baby Shoes
and mother of Dylan, age 3
California

It is important that when you start to gain weight, use Cocoa Butter Formula with Vitamin E on your stomach because it smoothes marks, tones skin, and reduces stretch marks.

Colleen, doctor of chiropractic and mother of Amelia, age 9 months
Colorado

A massage is not a luxury during pregnancy and your child's first year. Your child's health is directly related to your wellness. Receive massages at least once a month during your pregnancy and the first few months after delivery to keep your immune system in peak performance to help your body adjust to dramatic physical changes.

Aimee, certified pre/postnatal and infant massage therapist
Illinois

This is the one time in your life when it is in your best interest (and your child's) to care for and pamper yourself. Take it seriously. Nap, get a foot massage, simplify your schedule, eat well, and do things you love.

Jesse, childbirth educator, birth doula, and mother of Dashiell, age 1
Oregon

If you're pregnant, you've probably heard of toxoplasmosis because it can cause serious birth defects. Being pregnant does not mean you have to give up living with and caring for your beloved cat. Toxoplasmosis is easily avoided by practicing good hygiene and responsible pet care. Avoid handling or eating uncooked meat. Keep your cat safely indoors and away from wildlife. Have someone else clean the litter box daily. If you must clean the litter box, wear rubber gloves and thoroughly wash your hands afterward. Feed cats only commercially prepared cat food.

Martha Jones, editor of www.therealmartha.com
Missouri

During your pregnancy, sleep, sleep, sleep and relax as much as possible. And get those pampering treatments in now — manicures, pedicures, haircuts — because there's not as much time for it afterward.

Dawn, flight attendant gone insurance specialist and mother of
Madison Carmela, age 30 months

Sleep is not optional. Get as much as you need.

Susan Gmeiner, president of Maya Wrap and mother of
Arj, age 14, Michael, age 12, and Karl, age 4
North Carolina

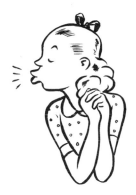

Sex Stuff

You can not poke your baby's head. You can not crush, jostle, or otherwise harm your baby by having relations while you are pregnant. But you may have to find new positions, locations, or even endure a kick or a poke reminding you that you are no longer alone anymore!

Jennifer, stay-at-home wife and mother of Magolia, age 4, and Van Royal, age 2
Utah

Every man fears for some reason that when making love to his pregnant wife, the head of the baby may be poked by him during intercourse. Reassure him that this is not possible! He should rest at ease that the baby will never know what is going on. Most likely the baby will sleep during the rocking motion.

Gina, banker and mother of Amanda, age 8, and Lilli, age 2
Florida

Get creative, connect, and have fun. You might not have the bed to yourselves again for a long while! And if you really don't feel up to the whole sha-bang, be sure to be affectionate, hug a lot, and "make out" as much as possible!

Danielle, nurse practitioner and mother of Gillian, age 6
Montana

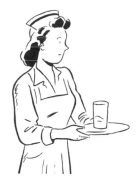

—Choosing Health Care—

Use a nurse midwife! They will work to make your birth the experience you wish it to be. They take time to get to know you, listen to your concerns, and provide the level of support you need – all within a safe and caring environment. You can labor without medication or with an epidural. And afterwards, you will feel like your birth was the special event it was meant to be.

**Ronni, nurse midwife and mother of Isaac, age 4, and Emmett, age 2
Pennsylvania**

Get a second opinion! Don't always take your doctor's word for it. He may be biased to one certain thing. I was told to have a C-section because I was "too small" for the baby to fit. After much research and several other opinions, we chose a midwife. At 42 weeks I gave birth to a 10-pound baby boy, vaginally, in my own home! Since then I have had three more babies (all big ones!) at home and in the water. I am SO GLAD I didn't take the first option I heard but researched and made the right decision for us. I found out that the doctor who told me to have a C-section tells almost every woman that, and he has an unusually high C-section rate.

**Tiffany, childbirth educator, doula, wife, and mother of
Ethan, age 7, Kellen, age 4, Tarin, age 3, and Presley, age 8 months
Georgia**

Many first-time moms are afraid to choose a midwife and opt for the more traditional OB. I would strongly recommend checking into using a midwife. Have a least one meeting with one to get your questions answered. There are many misconceptions out there, and if you can be open-minded, you will find that midwives offer a nice alternative to traditional OB care. I did so with both my children and had a wonderful experience.

Tari, mother of Grant, age 10, and Anthony, age 2
Pennsylvania

It is okay to switch health care providers, even in the eighth month, if you feel uncomfortable with the philosophy of your current provider. Having a positive birth experience is the bottom line, and that usually happens when mom feels as though she has some control over her birth experience. If your provider isn't open to at least some of your wishes, then you are less likely to come away feeling good about your birth experience. Whether you view the birth of your child as positive or negative can be reflected in feeding, parenting, and self-esteem issues.

Ann Israel, Lamaze certified birth educator, certified prenatal yoga teacher, and mother of Ben, age 12, and Stephen, age 10
Maryland

Interviewing my primary care person before taking her on was the greatest asset to me. (I interviewed four home birth midwives.) First, decide on the place you want to birth (hospital, birth center, home), then find the midwife who supports you in this and your other views about giving birth.It is critical for you to feel comfortable and in control because once in labor, you are no longer truly in control, for that is all about letting go!

Diane Hynes, shiatsu/craniosacral practitioner and mother of Taegan, age 28 months
New Jersey

Choose someone you trust. If the OB/Dr. doesn't take the time to talk with you and answer your questions, then find a new one! Don't stay with someone you don't trust! Moms know best — trust your instincts!

Trisha, stay-at-home mother of Emily Faith, age 8 months
Manitoba, Canada

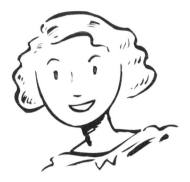

Doulas

During your pregnancy, hire a doula! Doulas can provide support before and after the birth as well as during. It's extra support and nurturing for the mom and her partner during their transition into parenthood. A doula can help a woman feel empowered to make choices, and we all know that moms always have lots of choices to make!

Lori, childbirth and breastfeeding educator and mother of Elizabeth, age 19, Isabella, age 5, and Zain, age 4
Missouri

Get a doula! She will make all the difference when it comes to helping you have a safe, fulfilling birth free from medical intervention. With my first baby (now 14), I used a doula. With my second baby (now 7), I did not. My first was born with no medical interventions (not even an IV) and was delivered in nine hours. My second baby was intervention, and it took me 24 hours of labor with her. I thought I knew what to ask and the alternatives that could help me; but when you're in "that space of birthing," getting facts and information aren't always at the top of your list, and my husband was so upset about my difficulties…he was no help. We needed someone to advocate for us. When I share birth experiences, I gleefully express my joy over my first birth and usually skim over my second.

JaLynn, mother of Kassie, age 14, and Kayla, age 7
Michigan

Get a doula! Hiring a doula was the best money we spent in the whole pregnancy/birth/early infancy period. A doula is a childbirth coach who not only will know everything there is to know about childbirth, but someone who will stay with you during your labor, unlike most doctors or nurses. Doulas don't intervene in the birth or get in the way of the OB, midwife, or nurses, but they will hold your hand (or your husband's), help you remember to breathe, and help you make decisions based on what you'd planned on before the pain and anxiety of actual labor set in. If I hadn't had a doula for my first son (my second is adopted), I know I would have had all sorts of interventions, probably been induced, and may have ended up having a C-section. Each of these things is sometimes medically necessary, of course, but I was able to avoid them because I had my doula by my side the whole time. As it turned out, my first son was my one-and-only birth experience; and thanks to my doula, it turned out great.

Adrienne Ehlert Bashista, author of *When I Met You*, a story of Russian adoption, and mother of Jacob, age 5, and Jamie, age 2
North Carolina

I could write a whole chapter on doulas! The best place to find a doula is at www.dona.org. Mothers-to-be should expect a doula to listen, first and foremost. The doula that talks too much is usually not overly helpful. Mothers need to talk and express their hopes and dreams, their fears and concerns. The doula's job is to listen with compassion, not to fix the problems or take them away; to acknowledge the mother and allow her the space to explore her feelings and figure out ways of coping. Mothers should expect their choices in childbirth to be honored. They should expect discretion and confidentiality. They should not expect clinical care. They should feel safe with the doula, and there should be a positive emotional connection. I like to say that when I feel I could crawl into someone's lap and cry if I needed to, then that's complete support to me! Most doulas provide one or two prenatal visits in the mother's home, phone support during pregnancy, continuous presence during labor and birth (which includes massage, help with positions and breathing, encouraging words, information/translation of medical terms as necessary), and one or two postpartum visits. Most doulas usually stay about an hour postpartum and help the mother wanting to breastfeed to put the baby to the breast. My doulas provide a written account of the birth for the mother, although this is not a standard practice nationwide.

Ilana Stein, doula trainer and mentor and childbirth educator
New York

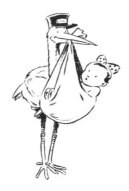

Birth Options

If you want a natural setting where you can be more in control, try checking into a free-standing birth center. These incredible birth centers are now providing beautiful births in many states of our country and can often be found on the Web site www.nacc.org, which is the National Association of Childbearing Centers. As a doula I hear and read about women who want to have the homey environment and low interventions but aren't quite ready to go the more radical home birth route. A birth center is the perfect solution. They are in close proximity for the rare transport to the hospital and usually feature both midwives and one or more OB's dedicated to unmedicated, noninterventive births. I tell you this as one who experienced all three settings: hospital, birth center, and, finally, home birth. I believe midwifery to be the best care possible and an out-of-hospital setting the ideal. Have a wonderful birth!

Kristin, mother of Kaitlin, age 9, Jacob, age 7, and Reilly, age 3 months
Vermont

Don't be afraid to try something different. We decided against the "traditional classes" and took HypnoBirthing. It was the greatest experience, and it allowed us to have a natural birth for our first beautiful child. If you want to bring your baby into the world without stress and the use of pain medications, this is a fantastic practice. Not only did I learn more about my unborn child and her needs, but I also learned more about my body, what it is capable of, and how to have a wonderful birth experience.

Heather, mother of Amelia, age 2 months
Wisconsin

If it makes sense, have your baby at home with a trained, experienced midwife. Home birth provides safe, customized, continuous, compassionate, peaceful care for mom and baby.

Joyce, midwife, doula, and mother of
David, age 9 and hospital born, and Julia, age 5 and born at home
Massachusetts

Look into home birth as an option. There are many studies published on the safety of home birth. Hospital birth is not always the safest option. Home birth allows MUCH more freedom and options. It's YOUR birth, no theirs.

Emily
Oregon

Pain control is all about mind control. Hypnobirthing classes and hypnosis therapy was extremely helpful in gaining control over those thoughts and feelings that can make you tense and thus make labor more uncomfortable. I was able to labor at home and deliver drug free with my first child.

Kathleen, homemaker and mother of Mary Elizabeth, age 6 months
New Mexico

If you are trying to decide whether or not to have an epidural, try not to make that decision based on the assumption that you are incapable of having an unmedicated birth experience! I had a home birth, and the thing that got me though the contractions was the idea that pain is only pain, nothing more, nothing less. Don't be afraid of it. Plenty of women have little or no pain during childbirth, and how will you know if you are one of them if you don't try? Humans, especially women, can withstand enormous amounts of discomfort and pain. You can do it!

Susan, mother of Athena, age 16 months
Colorado

Be proactive in your health care: research, research, research! Many standard medical protocols are not based on research but rather malpractice insurance protocols. What they provide as "options" may not truly be your only choices.

Emily
Oregon

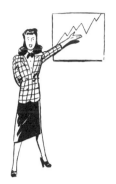

Birthing Plans

Try not to be too influenced by others telling you how to give birth. This is a chance to be a "team" with your unborn child. It is your opportunity to do something really important together. Make a birth plan that suits the both of you, not something fear-based or what others say for you to do. It is distressing how much focus is on the pain of childbirth and not on the incredible empowering experience it can be. I had both of my children at home, and those were the two best days of my life. I wouldn't have traded a moment of either experience for all the epidurals and ease in the world. I think that fear robs us of an authentic experience. However, just because I had my children at home does not mean that I think every woman should so this. I just think that as mothers we need to take responsibility for our own birth experiences for ourselves and for our children.

**Catherine, business owner and mother of Dylan, age 16, and Will, age 13
Colorado**

It's great to be informed about the facility you are going to give birth in and the types of procedures to expect. It is more important to keep an open mind and listen to the medical professionals. They have you and your baby's best interest at heart, or they should. When you plan too much, things do not go according to plan. Keep an open mind.

**Dawn, RN, and mother of Sophia, age 3, and Analiese, age 1
New Jersey**

You are in control of this pregnancy and birth. You hire the care provider: they work for you. But in labor, it's all about having been in control to this point in order to give it up. The trust and security you have developed with your care provider allows you the freedom to let go now. Laboring and giving birth are kin to good sex. You must be able to entrust yourself to your surroundings in order to release control and give your body into the process. TIP: Find the care provider and birth setting that you feel comfortable and safe with.

Rebecca, midwife and mother of Russell, age 22 (hospital born), Jamie, age 19 (home born unattended), Sterling, age 17 (home born unattended), and Elizabeth, age 11 (midwife attended home birth)
Kansas/California

You have it in your head how things should be before, during, and after the birth. Don't let anyone tell you that their "rules" won't accommodate your desires if they are reasonable enough. I've had to stand up to nurses who wanted to take my baby to the nursery, doctors who wanted to wake my sleeping newborn at midnight to finish the exam they didn't have time for earlier (therefore leaving me, a sleeping new mother, with an irate newborn), and all sorts of rules that can be bent, if not broken, if you complain enough. Remember always that this is your birth, your baby, and frankly, you're the customer, and the customer is always right. Stand up for what you want.

Jennifer, accountant and mother of
Alex, age 9, Veronica, age 4, and Matthew, age 2
Minnesota

Giving birth to your baby naturally or not is a personal choice. Do your homework so you know about standard procedures, medications, and interventions. Create a birth plan by at least your seventh month and have it approved by both your OB and pediatrician. Keep a signed copy with you, just in case your doctors are not on call for the birth.

Jennifer, stay-at-home mother of Milo, age 15 months
Illinois

If you plan to have a hospital birth, get a midwife, doula, or someone who has had a baby to stay with you at home as long as you can. Your chances for a good natural birth are better than going early to hospital.

Ezelda, midwife and mother of Themis, age 3 and born at home
EEC, Greece

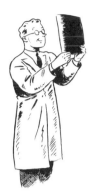

— Prenatal Test Anxiety —

The worst experience of my pregnancy was getting the results from the quad screen blood test and finding out that I had "screened positive" for Downs. I was incredibly worried, and it was all for nothing. The doctor failed to tell me that I would automatically screen positive because of my age until after I took the test [amino], so the test [blood] was inconclusive, the worry was unnecessary, and it was all avoidable if she has just told me in advance. Her response was, "Well, you're having an amino so you'll know definitely then." Yeah, the amino was a few weeks later, and you then have to wait for the results. I ended up having a healthy baby, but I could have been spared the weeks of worry and stress. I won't have the blood test next time and will just have the amino.

Elisa, management consultant and mother of Quinn, age 17 months
Colorado

Keep your pregnancy as natural as possible!! Keep away from ultrasounds!! We don't really know the effect on our growing babies. Ultrasound was invented to detect war ships. Now it's used much too often to scan a growing fetus. If you are a normal, healthy, pregnant woman, trust your body and God to let your baby grow as he/she should!!

Ezelda, midwife and mother of Themis, age 3 and born at home
EEC, Greece

Before you have any testing done for genetic diseases, please discuss with your partner first what you would do if something came back positive. What you would do can decide whether or not you will even get the tests done.

**Wendy, counselor and mother of Katie, age 15 months,
and expecting Baby #2 in April
New Jersey**

Genetic counseling is a relatively new field. A skilled genetic counselor is trained to help you sort through the risks specific to you and help you consider your options. Psychologically, women make different choices based on their personal beliefs, their perception of their own risks, the accuracy of the tests involved, and their perception of their ability to cope with a potential special needs child.

For most women, the reason to use this earlier detection test is psychological. Should they receive bad news, terminating a pregnancy before 12 weeks looms less traumatic. And shortening the period of emotional stress caused by "not knowing" if everything is all right may play a factor in women who are at greater risk of abnormalities due to family medical history.

Like any other parenting decision that will arise in the future, the answer that is right for you is the one you make together. Be prepared to reach out for help along the way, especially if your genetic test comes back positive. Genetic counselors and family therapist experts in the prenatal period and parenting fields can support you in working through the emotional repercussions to the choices medical science has now made available to us.

What is the "right" choice, however, is personal. And our decision shapes not only our lives, but the lives of our family members, too. For some the answer of whether to test is an easy one; for others, not. But when a test comes back with possibilities for genetic problems, the choices get harder for almost everyone. With choice comes responsibility and commitment to that choice. With commitment comes maturity. Prenatal testing can introduce a course of soul-searching. But isn't that what parenthood requires?

**Gayle Peterson, MSSW, LCSW, Ph. D., family therapist specializing in prenatal and family development (www.askdrgalye.com), author of *Making Healthy Families* and *An Easier Childbirth*, advisory board member for *Fit Pregnancy* magazine, mother of two adult children, and a proud grandmother
California**

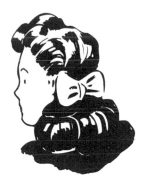

— Complications and Loss —

Get any suspected miscarriages verified by a doctor. If you have
multiple miscarriages, many doctors will not run tests unless you've
had two or three confirmed miscarriages. In addition, mothers
trying after miscarriages need to stand up for themselves and
remember that the doctor is working for them, not the other way
around. Do not hesitate to get second, third, fourth, or even fifth
opinions if a doctor is not working for you.

**Krissi, mother of Madeleine, age 19 months
California**

Don't let any medical procedures (D&C) take away the wonder of
"giving birth" to your small embryo/fetus at home and saying
goodbye to your little one who was never meant to grow full term
but was given to you to appreciate your living children and to count
the many blessings God gives us every day!

**Ezelda, midwife and mother of Themis, age 3 and born at home
EEC, Greece**

If you want a vaginal birth but your baby is breech, discuss a procedure
called an "external version" with your care provider. The success rate is
good, and complications are rare if you turn out to be a candidate for it.

**Annmarie, attorney and mother of Eve, age 3, and Nathaniel, age 4 months
New Jersey**

I was so impressed with the Prenatal Cradle. I was shocked to learn that the pain I was feeling at 16 weeks was due to strained ligaments. It seemed too early in the pregnancy to be dealing with this. My doctor told me to get the Prenatal Cradle, and I am so glad that I did. Within two days of wearing the product the pain had disappeared! I have been wearing the Prenatal Cradle for three happy weeks and am able to work and exercise in it. I barely notice I'm wearing it. I am very thankful for the product and so glad that I didn't waste my time and money with the cheap department store maternity belts. The phone staff was very friendly and helpful. My only wish is that the Prenatal Cradle was easier to find in stock in my area.

Heather
Georgia

Many women have major hip pain during pregnancy. Some women actually have to sit in a wheelchair during their late pregnancy, and some are stuck in a wheelchair AFTER their pregnancy as well (some for many years!).

The main issue is to look after yourself, and take this very seriously. Be very careful with what you do. Exercise can very often make things much worse. Be careful doing housework, and be careful walking up stairs. When you walk, take small steps. During my second pregnancy I had to use crutches some weeks to get around in my house, and at night I could hardly get out of bed when going to the toilet. It hurt so very much! I tried going for walks outside, but after about 50 meters my only thought was "how on earth am I going to get back home again......."

Be careful, and let your husband, family, or friends do the heavy work and housework around the house! Please listen, or else you might have problems for the rest of your life! Still today, I have a lot of pain in my right hip — especially if I lie down on a hard flat floor, hard mattress, or similar. I can hardly get up again. At night I usually put a pillow under me knee or between me legs — it gives good support and helps relieve the pain.

Here, in Norway, hip pain is actually a BIG problem during pregnancy, and there is an organization for women with hip pain during pregnancy. Awareness is growing among doctors and nurses. In the USA, there seems to be little knowledge about the suffering that many women experience during pregnancy due to hip pain. So if your doctor tells you that you complain to much, you should not listen too closely because so many doctors seem to be ignorant of this problem. This is a topic that should be much more focused on by doctors.

Kathrine Jölle Wathne, owner of www.babysite.org, and mother of
Dina Kamilla, age 10, and Herman Andre, age 7
Norway

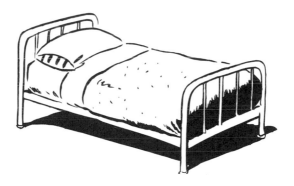

Being on Bed Rest

These four things were really helpful for dealing with bed rest.

1. Try to stick to a schedule, and try to be showered and dressed every day before noon. Just having a routine will help your day go quicker and will help life seem more normal.

2. Do as much as the doctors will allow you to (but no more than that). My doctors let me have a recumbent stationary bike, and I was allowed to ride it two times a day for 20 minutes. I was also allowed to be upright for 15 to 20 minutes every 2 to 3 hours as long as I didn't walk too far, and I took advantage of that as much as I could.

3. Get out of the house as much as possible. During Christmas season my husband would drive me around for a little while to look at the lights, or we'd go someplace where he'd be able to push me in a wheel chair. Just to leave the house and see people was a great thing. It will make you feel more plugged in to the rest of the world.

4. Stay mentally active. I got so many great gifts when I was on bed rest...puzzle books, knitting and art kits, books in general. Anything that is engaging and will help pass the time is great.

Kelly, mother of Matthew, age 4 months
New Jersey

During my second pregnancy, I was placed on bed rest due to premature labor. I had somehow pictured bed rest as a lengthy time of being in bed while I worked diligently on a laptop, got caught up on my writing, and relaxed. Unfortunately, my idea was far from reality. I spent four weeks lying on my left side (I'm left-handed, so writing was out), reading and watching television. I was allowed to get up to go to the bathroom and to sit up only to eat. It was a great challenge for me, a person who loves activity, works from home, and has a toddler! I realized though that I actually was luckier than some, and that what I was doing was very important for my baby.

Some days I felt great. Some days I felt depressed. Most days I felt pretty useless. There were several things I did to help me get through this period. First I focused on how important this was for my baby. I took it one day at a time and considered each day a gift to my baby. I would tell myself that this wasn't about me but about him, and I wouldn't suffer any ill effects, though he should reap great rewards by being able to be near to full term. I also kept an ultrasound picture next to me on my end table of "essentials." Whenever I felt down, I would look at Jack's picture and think about how he was still in me, developing.

Another thing I did was to take up any friend's offers of help. For probably the first time in my life whenever anyone said, "Is there anything I can do?" I said, "Yes!" My parents and mother-in-law were tag-teaming staying with us to care for our one-year-old and to take care of my needs, but if anyone offered to run an errand, bring a meal, come and visit, or take my daughter on a walk, I said, "Yes!"

I tried, too, not to let my mind get inactive. Being on bed rest gave me plenty of time to worry about various things, from the baby's development to my daughter (who couldn't understand why Mommy was lying around all the time and not taking care of her), to work left undone, etc. I love to read, and I did so for hours each day. I had my husband bring me things to read and learn about (the Greek alphabet, my old Italian books, British history, art magazines, etc.). I watched lots of the Olympics coverage as well, though I stayed away from depressing movies, scary true birth stories, and often, the news!

I focused each day on how this was temporary. The end would come, and then I'd have a beautiful baby. My husband cheered me on, saying how only I could do this for Jack and how important I was. I ignored insensitive remarks from people who responded that bed rest "must be nice" since they were so busy all the time. I prayed each day for the strength that I needed and for my family.

And finally, the end came! I had made it! When I reached 35 weeks, I turned to my husband and said, "Well, now, that wasn't so bad!" and he just smiled and responded, "I love your 'pregnancy amnesia'!"

**Dr. Beth, developmental psychologist and educator and mother of
Anne, age 1 and Jack, age 1 month
Massachusetts**

Whatever you do when on bed rest for months during pregnancy, eat very light because the weight will be hard to take off, especially when you're older and decide to have children.

Regina, buyer/purchaser and mother of
Ronald, age 24, Elijah, age 11, and Ajhand, age 2
New Jersey

While you are on bed rest, you are doing the most important job of your life. Every day counts: do not lose sight of that.

Alexandra, mother of Chloe, age 2 and expecting Baby #2 in January
Pennsylvania

When the doctor puts you on bed rest, DO IT!

Mary, professor and mother of Sean, age 10 months
Illinois

Don't think about the weeks or months ahead. Instead, focus on that week, that day, that hour, that minute – however small you have to break it down. This is your big chance to practice living in the moment.

Moira, HypnoBirthing practitioner and mother of
Calum, age 5, and Isobel, age 2
British Columbia, Canada

I was very upset when my doctor placed me on hospital bed rest. Thankfully, I had a very loving and supporting family who was there with me the entire time to help me through it. My husband and close friends frequently brought my two older children to visit and helped them maintain their normal routine in my absence. My husband also bought me stationary so that I could write cute little letters to my children reminding them that I loved them, and I would be home as soon as I could. It was adorable when I finally came home and saw all of my letters to them proudly displayed on the refrigerator. I also kept a private journal for myself to let out some of my feelings and deal with my changing emotions. My family brought me many books to read as well. But the one thing that really helped me through it was their constant presence and the knowledge that I was doing the right thing for my growing baby.

Katherine, stay-at-home mother of
Tim, age 9, Nicole, age 6, and Jennifer, age 1½
West Virginia

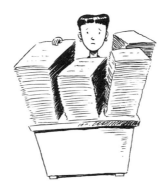

Work Issues

Know your rights during pregnancy and parenthood. Find out as much as possible about what you are personally entitled to because many of the benefits vary based on the length of your employment, who you work for, and where you live. You can contact your Human Resources manager, Personnel manager, trade union representative, or your local job center or benefits agency to learn more about what you can expect. Also, use the internet to research current legislation. Knowing the laws that affect you will help you stand up for yourself and protect your rights.

You are not legally obligated to tell your employer that you are expecting until you are ready to do so. Once you choose to tell your boss your news, you may be entitled to special rights like time off for prenatal care, health and safety protection, and protection from dismissal or unfair treatment because of your pregnancy. Decide when and how you want to share your news. It's usually best to request a meeting at a time when your boss is reasonably relaxed and receptive. Realize that although your boss may be delighted for you, your pregnancy poses many challenges for him. Work with your boss to alleviate concerns.

**Natalie Gahrmann, author of *Succeeding as a SuperBusy Parent*,
life and parent coach, and mother of two
New Jersey**

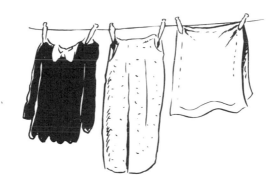

Maternity Clothes

Maternity clothes should make you feel pretty and be fun, while at the same time show off your biggest, new asset! While shopping, keep in mind: if it looks like maternity wear, leave it on the rack. Choose pieces that look like your pre-pregnancy clothes and will leave your friends wondering if they come in regular sizes, too!

**Sheryl Fernandez, owner of Bellies and Bubbles Maternity
and mother of Dalton, age 16 months
Pennsylvania**

Buy one or two really nice maternity outfits and wear them all the time.

**Raya, owner of www.roundbelly.com, and mother of
Galen, age 5, Ewan, age 3, Ian, age 1, and expecting another
Minnesota**

Do not give away or pack away your maternity clothes at the end of your pregnancy. You can plan to still need to wear you maternity pants for at least a couple more months. Going home in your pre-pregnancy clothes is a cruel myth.

**Leigh Donadieu, publisher of *Cuizine* magazine and mother of
Mitchell, age 4, and Ruth, age 2
New Jersey**

With my second pregnancy, I discovered underbelly jeans. They are the most comfortable pants for the entire pregnancy, and I'm still wearing them two months postpartum. They look like normal jeans, but they stretch and don't have a zipper. They do have pockets and a wide, covered elastic waist. No one can tell that they are maternity pants. I got mine at Babystyle. I also recommend drawstring pants for the first few months of pregnancy (and postpartum) when hips expand, but not the belly. They also fit under a growing belly and are very comfortable and stylish.

Liza, stay-at-home mother of Anna Lucy, age 2, and Francis, age 8 weeks
Colorado

Once your clothes start getting tight, go out and buy yourself a couple pairs of your favorite jeans two sizes larger than usual…you will feel much happier and thinner! You can extend their life by looping a rubber band through the button hole to expand the waistband. These jeans will be great for the first couple of months postpartum when you don't want to try on your old clothes. Who feels great slopping around in sweatpants all the time?

Pat McGough-Wujcik, drummer for The Mydols, an all-mom band and mother of
Megan, age 19, Nick, age 12, Ryan, age 10, and Sophy, age 4
Michigan

Maternity clothes are so expensive, and you only wear them for a few months. I never had a hard time finding them in cheap thrift stores. I found good quality clothes even for my twin pregnancy (when I needed a 3X). I then sold them on eBay at profit when I was finished with them.

Elyssia, professional mother of
Samantha, age 8, Sophia, age 3, and Thomas and Iris, age 1

Don't spend a ton of money on maternity wear, because you won't be wearing it for that long. Stores like Target, The Gap, and Old Navy carry affordable, stylish, maternity wear. If possible, also try to inherit some cute items from friends who have recently been pregnant. And steal from your husband! Don't sacrifice your style just because you're pregnant, but try not to spend a lot of money either. Save the big shopping trip for after your birth when you're celebrating the first day you fit back into your pre-pregnancy jeans!

Lorraine, hair stylist and mother of Taylor
California

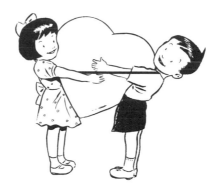

Boy or Girl?

With my first pregnancy, I was torn between wanting to know the sex of my baby and not wanting to know until the baby's birth. Lucky for me, I ran into a friend who helped me decide not to find out the baby's sex before birth. She described my baby inside of me as a beautifully wrapped package, a gift to me, a special surprise that I was not supposed to peak at. I loved the idea of waiting to open my present – waiting for the day the gift is given to me through labor. It was the right decision for my family with both of my births. The anticipation and excitement surrounding both of my daughters' births was so much fun!

Candace, The Bradley Method Childbirth Educator and stay-at-home mother of Perry Elizabeth, age 5, and Zoe Adair, age 18 months
Texas

I felt I could really identify with my baby once I knew what the sex was. As far as being surprised or having nothing left to be excited about, we decided not to pick a definite name until we saw him. And believe me, when you see your baby for the first time, it doesn't matter if you've known the sex all along; it is still the most amazing and wonderful experience of your life.

Kara, mother of Kyle, age 11 months
New Jersey

My one biggie is not to go out and do any gender specific decorating or clothes shopping unless the sex has been confirmed via amnio, as ultrasounds are NOT 100% accurate, no matter if the technicians are seeing male or female genitalia! It's nice to have a good guess, but it's only a good guess, and people need to remember that.

**Debbie, owner www.coconutbeach.com, and mother of
CJ, age 6½, and Rachel, age 2
New Jersey**

I recently gave birth to my first child, and my husband and I decided not to find out the gender. There are certainly disadvantages to that method—having to refer to the baby as "it" or "he/she" and not knowing what color clothes to buy or how to decorate the nursery—but the joys of waiting outweighed the minor hassles. If I had known whether I was having a boy or a girl, I would have missed out on the fun of hearing people's predictions. Everyone from my mother to the cashier at the grocery store guessed what I would have. (It turns out that the cashier was right!) Even more importantly, though, not knowing whether the baby would be a boy or a girl got me through the last moments of a long and difficult labor. The pushing phase was exhausting, and it took every ounce of energy I had to get through it. The anticipation and excitement of discovering whether I was giving birth to a daughter or a son gave me the impetus I needed to keep going.

**Cathy, mother of Maggie, age 5 weeks
Ohio**

For your first baby let it be a surprise. It is a great feeling and a great surprise when you don't know what the sex of the baby is until you have him or her.

**Michelle, physical therapy aide and mother of Robert, age 5
New Jersey**

I decided to find out my baby's sex before the birth. I liked the idea of being able to choose a single name, start decorating the nursery, and begin buying gender specific clothing right away. It saved me a lot of stress after the birth, because my baby already had lots of clothing, and her nursery was set up perfectly for a little girl.

**Lorraine, hair stylist and mother of Taylor
California**

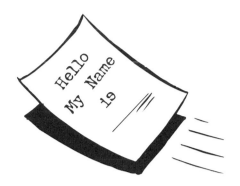

Choosing Names

"Try out" your baby's name for at least a few days. When you're talking about the baby, use the chosen name. "Sidney's kicking me," "Sidney and I are going for a walk," "Sidney, clean up your room." If you're tired of the baby's name after a few days, then that's NOT the name you should choose. Move on to the next name.

**Sherry Bonelli, www.PregnancyStore.com, and mother of
Connor, age 6, and twins Sidney and Kiley, age 2
Illinois**

My children's names were created. They are a combination of my name and their dad's name (Melanie and Donnell).

**Melanie, full-time domestic engineer, educator, author, and mother of twins
Meldonár and Meldoníque
Massachusetts**

When we chose Emily's name, I had to make sure it flowed with her brothers' names. So I practiced calling them in for dinner by quietly yelling, "Sam, Michael, Emily, it's time for dinner!" The name just fit right in!

**Jennifer, educator and mother of
Samuel, age 12, Michael, age 7, and Emily, age 4
New Jersey**

Wait until AFTER you have definitely decided on a name before telling people. Don't ask opinions. Once you have decided, tell people this IS his/her name, leaving no room for further discussion.

Margaret, homemaker and mother of Braden, age 4
Texas

Get your older children involved in the process of naming the new baby. The more they get involved in all sorts of preparations for the new arrival, the more excited (and less jealous) they'll be. Start building positive bonds among your children in the months leading up to the birth.

Barbara Freedman-De Vito, author and artist at Baby Bird Productions Children's Stories and Fairy Tales, www.babybirdproductions.com
Massachusetts

Don't follow the trend regarding the most popular baby names of the time. You don't have to name your baby something "cool" simply because that's what Madonna named her daughter or "Emily" because that's the most popular name at the time. There are a lot of "Britney's" out there! And remember that a name that sounds "creative" or "different" to you might just be just plain "weird" to someone else, and you and your child are going to be living with that name for a long time. Give your child a name that you and your husband both love, not one that you copied from a trend book or celebrity or the newspaper.

Emma, guidance counselor and mother of Drew, age 2
Louisiana

Deciding on a name for your future child is a very personal experience for you and your husband. While you don't have to ignore the advice of others around you, remember that you don't necessarily have to consider it either. Listen to what ideas your family and friends may have but, ultimately, choose a name that you and your husband both feel comfortable with. Don't be pressured into naming your son after your great-uncle if you don't want to. This is your child, and you and your husband have the right to name him/her whatever you wish. You may regret naming your son Sam if you knew you always wanted a Jared.

Suzanne, teacher and mother of Sean, age 19, and Jennifer, age 14
New Jersey

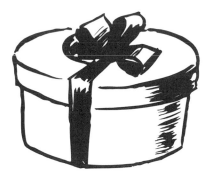

Registering for Gifts

Becoming new parents, we all want to buy all the latest and greatest baby items that we think we will need. But what I've found is that more times than not, you end up returning the product to the store because it really didn't fit your needs. Case in point: With my first born, I registered for a deluxe model high chair. I received the high chair but didn't use it for five months, so it sat in a box taking up space until I needed it; and then when I did put it together, the high chair was too high up. When we ate dinner, the baby was a foot taller than the rest of us. Feeding him was pretty difficult. I decided to buy a portable high chair that fit in a regular chair, and it worked perfectly and was more convenient than the large high chair. This was something that I would have never known as a first time parent. My advice: think before you buy. Does a friend or family member have what it is you're contemplating buying? If so, borrow and don't buy. Babies grow too fast, and before you know it, it will be time to invest in a toddler gadget.

Jenny Lovins, professional organizer, author of *Unclutter Your Life*, and mother of Jacob, age 5, and Grace, age 2
Virginia

When using a baby registry, don't pick out a cute diaper bag. Go for the more masculine "backpack" type so that Daddy doesn't feel uncomfortable taking the baby out alone. It also makes Dad feel more proud to hold it when it isn't so cutesy.

Heidi, teacher and mother of Elisabeth, age 4, and Lauren, age 2
California

Take an experienced friend with you when you register to help pick out items rather than doing it blindly with your significant other.

Heidi, teacher and mother of Elisabeth, age 4, and Lauren, age 2
California

Ask for gift cards and then buy diapers!

Meredith, marketing consultant and mother of Eliza, age 3, and Zachary, age 1½
New Jersey

If you have a two-story house, it is very useful to have two exersaucers and two swings. That way there's always a safe place to put the baby no matter where you are in the house.

Stacy, graphic artist, owner of Inkspot Creations, and mother of Julia, age 18 months
New Jersey

Don't forget to register for practical things like diapers, baby shampoo, formula, etc. Also, be sure to register for things for you as a parent, such as an extra cordless phone, film, or parenting books.

Kim Danger, owner www.mommysavers.com, and mother of
Sydney, age 5, and Nicholas, age 1
Minnesota

Talk to mothers before you register and see what items they feel are really useful. Investigate those products. Check for recalls and customer satisfaction. Go and try these things out in the stores before you make a final decision. So many products seem like a good idea but are not always necessary. Many things that I thought would make my life easier did not.

Dawn, RN, and mother of Sophia, age 3, and Analiese, age 1
New Jersey

You don't need every baby contraption. The stores can be daunting to a mother-to-be, but it doesn't make you a better parent the more gadgets you have. Go with your guts and your current lifestyle. Keep it somewhat simple so you can still cuddle and hold your baby who doesn't stay that way for very long.

Kim, mother of Elias, age 4, Rhett, age 2½, and Sloan, age 8 months
Arkansas

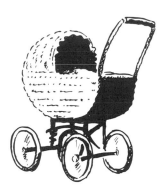

Equipment & Supplies

Invest money in a high quality baby swing with a silent battery-operated motor. Make sure it has a seat that holds an infant lying down, and make sure the seat can be removed and used as a carrier. Some even have a seat that can be used in the car! When I had Jimmy, I bought a cheap wind-up swing with a hard plastic seat designed for the baby to sit in – he couldn't lie down. Boy, did I regret it! The hand crank made noise when it was wound up, so just as Jimmy was falling asleep, the swing would lose power, and I'd have to crank it again. The cranking noise would always wake him up. Plus, if he did fall asleep I couldn't move him. Getting him out of the fixed seat was too difficult to do without waking him. Trust me. Buy a nice swing and save money elsewhere.

Mara, chemist and mother of Jimmy, age 10
Nevada

If there was one item that I felt I could not have done without in the first months, it would be the Boppy Pillow. It was obviously great for nursing. But other unexpected uses arose, including propping baby for family and friend viewings (especially if you didn't want everyone handling your newborn!). Putting baby on her tummy on the back of the "U" shape also gave her early use of her hands while on her tummy, and placing it on her hips when she was learning to sit up was a great way for her to find her balance without too many hard landings!

Kathleen, homemaker and mother of Mary Elizabeth, age 6 months
New Mexico

BEFORE you give birth, look into the perfect baby sling. The internet is a great place to search. Make sure you try it out before you buy it. Practice putting the sling on with a doll, stuffed animal, or bag of flour. Believe me, being at ease with a good sling will be invaluable after your baby is born when you want to be out and about getting things done. You can wear your baby, which he/she will love, and hardly have to slow down!

Kristin, mother of Conor, age 5 and born in a hospital, and Bella, age 7 months and born at home in the water Washington

According to the U.S. Consumer Product Safety Commission (CPSC), over 11,000 children are rushed to emergency rooms each year from injuries related to strollers. Carriers and car seats are the only juvenile products responsible for more injuries. Between 1990 and 2004, the CPSC has recalled over 23 different strollers because of injuries, product failures, or identified hazards. Get the list at www.KidsinDanger.org, or www.CPSC.gov. Do not use these products. Contact the manufacturer or CPSC at 1-800-638-2772 to find out how to comply with recalls. Be sure to return product registration cards so that the manufacturer can contact you directly in the case of a recall.

Nancy, child safety advocate and mother of Hannah, Lucy, and Walter Illinois

Some duplicates aren't necessarily a bad thing. We have two changing stations set up: the pack-n-play downstairs and a changing pad on a low dresser upstairs. Each has its own Diaper Genie. We also had a bouncy seat upstairs and one downstairs (one we registered for and received; the other was a hand-me-down). It saved us from running up and down the stairs or lugging heavy items back and forth.

Jennifer, editor and mother of Kayleigh, age 18 months Pennsylvania

Get a really firm pillow to rest your newborn on while he nurses. You need to hold the baby "up" to your breast rather than lean into him in order to prevent your back from becoming sore and stiff. The firm pillow allows baby to lie at the correct height, rather than be supported by mother's arms which quickly tire with a dozen feedings a day!

Sharon, stay-at-home mother of William, age 7, and Stephen, age 5 Illinois

A product called an Auto Mobile that attaches to the headliner of cars for infants in rear-facing car seats is a great idea! It keeps babies entertained while they are alone in the back seat. I saw it at my daughter-in-law's baby shower.

Ginny, retired and expecting grandmother of Parker or Paige
Texas

The most useful gift I have ever received was a pack of terry toweling nappies (diapers) when my first baby was born. They have so many uses: lie the baby on while changing nappies; mop up any accident; keep baby warm; use over your shoulder while burping the baby. I always have one by the crib to mop up any accidents at night and one in the car and the nappy bag. They wash really well and can be used over and over again, and they are relatively inexpensive. I am still using some of the same ones now for my fifth baby. The ones no longer used in the nursery have been used for wiping windows, etc.

Sian, clinical nurse specialist and mother of
Thomas, age 16, Chelsea, age 12, Courtney, age 11, Caprice, age 6, and Chanelle, age 1
Cheshire, United Kingdom

Buy some terry nappies (diapers) to use as bibs, pillow covers, shoulder covers for burping, etc.

Tamalyn Roberts, Web site owner, www.names2be.com, and mother of
Natalie, age 9, Matthew, age 7, and Paul, age 5
Anglesey, United Kingdom

Invest in a lightweight stroller to be kept in the car at all times. Be sure it has a tray so that baby may have a place for cup and snack. I liked Combi the best.

Angela, homemaker and mother of Dylan, age 10, and Nicholas, age 1½
California

A good baby carrier is one of the best investments you will make. An excellent resource is www.thebabywearer.com.

Susan Gmeiner, president of Maya Wrap and mother of
Arj, age 14, Michael, age 12, and Karl, age 4
North Carolina

I would love to advise all moms to begin bilingual instruction while they are pregnant through the use of my fun music CD's.

Beth Butler, founder of The BOCA BETH Program
Florida

Ask for a baby sling as a baby gift and ask an experienced mom to show you how to wear it. It allows baby to stay where he wants and needs to be – close to mother – while allowing you more freedom of movement and allowing you to quickly sense what your baby needs. You tune into each other, enabling you to catch his earliest cues of hunger, cold, etc. Babies are much more content and can use their energy for growth and development rather than fussing to get your attention so you can meet their needs.

Sharon, stay-at-home mother of William, age 7, and Stephen, age 5
Illinois

After my third child, I decided to do away with the baby monitor. Babies make sweet groans and grunts during their sleep which don't necessarily mean they are hungry or ready to get up. A baby monitor intensifies each noise, which makes mom get up even when she doesn't need to. Without a monitor, you will know when the baby really is ready to get up because he/she will be at a full cry and ready to eat. That way, baby won't fall asleep while trying to feed.

Cherie Drennan, lighting designer, www.heavenly-lights.com, and mother of
Johnny, age 12, Jordan, age 11, Olivia, age 9, Whit, age 7, and Gregory, age 3
Tennessee

The best piece of equipment I bought was my sling. The worst piece I bought was the crib…it's a very expensive toy chest.

Amanda, stay-at-home mother of Samantha Alexis, age 11 months
Ohio

Don't buy the huge high chairs that take up too much space. Instead, get the type that attaches to a chair and is portable and grows with the child. You remove the tray and use it as a booster seat as the child gets older.

Georgeanne, labor and postpartum doula and mother of
four and grandmother of four
Maryland

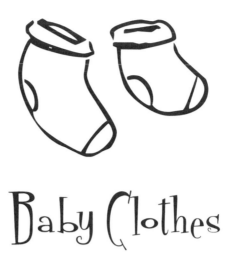

Baby Clothes

Instead of folding all of those new clothes you get for your newborn (and forgetting all about them until you find them by accident and your child is too big for them), hang them. Buy the small, baby-size hangers before you deliver and then hang the clothes up as you get them. You'll be able to see what you've got so much easier.

Andrea, public relations consultant and mother of Drew, age 11
Connecticut

I learned the hard way that when you get baby clothes for gifts, you should wash them before hanging them up or putting them away. When my son was born, I had all of these lovely clothes hanging up; and as I thought he'd fit into them, I'd put them on him, then wash them for next time. Well, I forgot that many clothes shrink when washed, so we had many clothes that were only worn once and then wouldn't fit again after washing.

Tania, labor doula and childbirth educator (CAPPA) and mother of
Stephen, age 13, Brendan, age 11, Kathryn, age 9, and Michael, age 7
Colorado

Use old diaper boxes to store either clothes the baby has grown out of or needs to grow in to. They are sturdy and in plentiful supply.

Jane, mother of Nicholas, age 3, and Sam and Will, age 16 months
New Jersey

Don't go through the trouble of buying a lot of newborn clothes because babies grow out of them way too fast. However, you really should buy at least one outfit that you really love to take to the hospital so the outfit your baby wears for his/her first official photo fits and really shows how big or small your baby is. You'll want to preserve this, and a baggy 0-3-month outfit just doesn't cut it.

Angie, mother of Connor, age 6 months
Tennessee

Buy unisex clothing in the boys' section. Boys clothing is often more durable and will last longer when passed down to siblings. When buying baby clothes, don't forget eBay. You may be able to find gently used clothing for considerable savings. Search for clothing in lots to save even more money. Don't forget to factor in shipping costs and pay close attention to the seller's feedback profile.

Kim Danger, owner www.mommysavers.com, and mother of
Sydney, age 5, and Nicholas, age 1
Minnesota

You do not need to spend extra money on Dreft or any other special baby laundry detergent. Simply buy one of the many "free" brands – as in free of dyes, scents, etc.

Jane, mother of Nicholas, age 3, and Sam and Will, age 16 months
New Jersey

An over-the-door shoe organizer is great for organizing baby's things, such as combs and brushes, socks, shoes, and little toys. The little compartments are also great for storing whole outfits, making dressing baby much easier.

Kim Danger, owner www.mommysavers.com, and mother of
Sydney, age 5, and Nicholas, age 1
Minnesota

Take any and all baby clothes you can from friends or family. Kids can go through many outfits per day, and each one does not have to be an A+ outfit. They can make great outfits to keep in the car or diaper bag in case of "blow out" diapers that leave you in need of a new outfit.

Christine, full-time diva and mother of Julia, age 2½, and Olivia, age 6 months
New Jersey

— Surviving the Shower —

No matter how bloated and squat you feel at the end of your pregnancy, do not wear heels to your baby shower! I buckled on strappy sandals before my shower to try to "lengthen" my chunky water-retaining legs. After only 20 minutes of greeting guests, my sandals came off and for the rest of the shower, I became the old cliché — barefoot and pregnant.

Kate, advertising account supervisor and mother of Jackson, age 4 months
Pennsylvania

If you are well into your pregnancy, don't feel bad about being overwhelmed. Use the bathroom (that you frequently visit) to just sit and get your thoughts or emotions together. It can be very overwhelming.

Christine, full-time diva and mother of Julia, age 2½, and Olivia, age 6 months
New Jersey

Opening all those presents can be exhausting — both physically and mentally. Take a few minutes to get your bearings so you know not only where great-aunt Minnie is sitting but what she looks like! And take a few breaks to stand up and take a walk or bathroom break. Make sure you get a slice of your cake, too!

Connie, publisher and mother of Holden, age 3
New Jersey

My first baby came with a traditional shower. It had the requisite baby shower games like Guess Her Girth (meaning my waist size!), What Baby Food Flavor Is This?, and more. We also had the obligatory gift-opening hour where I had to open and "ooh and ahh" over each present. While the gifts were lovely, I kept thinking, "Nobody was talking about my impending birth" (and I really wanted to hear about other women's experiences); "Nobody was talking about what becoming a mother was like" (and since I was the first of all of my friends, at age 32, there was nothing forthcoming from my peers); "Nobody was talking about anything that related to the challenges/ wondrous moments/pain/excitement/etc., that lay ahead." Then, I got a bigger shock while in labor: I needed a caesarean section. As a woman who had total faith in her body's ability to do anything (including running marathons!), it had not even registered as a possibility in my world. Afterwards, I felt let down, angry, confused.

Well, almost two years to the day after my beautiful son was born, I was expecting my second baby. My wonderful book club sisters wanted to celebrate with me. When I firmly insisted no shower was expected or needed (any second time mom will tell you that more "stuff" is the LAST thing she needs), one of the women in my group suggested a Blessing Way Ceremony. Little did any of us know how life-changing this experience was to be for every woman in attendance!

The basic underlying philosophy of the Blessing Way is to acknowledge a life transition and to embrace it. A Birth Blessing Way ceremony honors a woman's rite of passage from maiden to mother. This element, the acknowledgement — completely out in the open — that the group is gathering to discuss the expectant mother, her fears, hopes, dreams, her impending birth experience and to share the labor stories of her "village of women" is the central difference from most showers. The focus is primarily on the expectant mother, not on the baby, for it is the mother-to-be who will need the love and support to successfully and happily enter this new phase of life. It is then, also, a celebration of womanhood and friendships. It is not materialistic. Guests agree that bringing a gift for a friend is a great deal easier than thinking of a blessing or well-wish for her. So here is your warning: Sharing heart-felt sentiments in a group is an extremely profound undertaking. We women have so much to give each other and the Blessing Way gives us the means through its rituals to connect to what was, what is, and what will be.

A Blessing Way can be hosted in a number of ways. It can be an alternative to a traditional baby shower, or it can be an enhancement to one. First time mothers may want or need both components while experienced mothers oftentimes prefer the stand-alone ceremony as acknowledgement of another pregnancy without the "fuss."

Stefany Koslow, A Blessing Way guide, www.ablessingway.com, and mother of Gabriel, age 5, and Lily, age 3
New Jersey

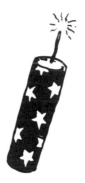

—Celebrating Pregnancy—

Do something special. Create a belly cast of your torso to commemorate your pregnancy. There are folks all over who can be hired to create your belly cast, or you can purchase a kit that will provide everything you need to create one with your partner, family, or at your baby shower.

Jala Smith, owner of Eternal Maternal
Oregon

Have your pregnant belly professionally photographed (my favorite pose – a close-up of my belly with my hands and my husband's hands resting on it). It's a unique and awesome keepsake of a remarkable time in your life.

Tammy, public relations manager and mother of
Lexi, age 9, Haylee, age 7, and Payton, due 11/23/04
Wisconsin

Cherish and preserve the look of your pregnant body by taking photos of yourself at all stages of your pregnancy. Be adventurous and bare as much as you feel comfortable with. I found it worth hiring a professional photographer to photograph the end of all "4" trimesters, the last including the baby herself in place of my belly. It can be very empowering to see yourself in this beautiful light.

Annmarie, attorney and mother of Eve, age 3, and Nathaniel, age 4 months
New Jersey

Time goes by waaaaaaaaaaay too fast. Take pictures and lots of them of your pregnancy, birth, and through the stages of your child's entire life. I know that along with these pictures it is a must to write down every little detail of babyhood that you want to remember. You will be amazed what special little details you will forget with time. Someday when you are reminiscing in your mind, it will bring a smile to your heart if you can read and remember these details of your little one. It will also be a treasure to your child when he/she grows up.

Lea, courtesy of The Center for Conscious Parenting, www.cfcp.info, mother of two little gems ages 3 and 2½ months
Oregon

Document everything from the moment you take a pregnancy test: your reaction to the pregnancy, your mate's reaction, the baby's heart rate the first time your hear it, your cravings, the emotions of pregnancy, choosing a name. Keep a journal and write letters to the baby. This will be such a precious gift to your child someday!

Jill, full-time mother of Alison, age 1
Illinois

Have your hubby or sibling or friend take a photo of you the same time each month. I did this with my best friend. The first week of every month we stood on her landing and took a front, side, and silly shot of her. At the end of the pregnancy you will be glad you have these. Although the pregnancy can seem like it's lasting forever at times, I don't know one woman who has ever had enough photo's of herself carrying the beautiful child she now has.

Christine, full-time diva and mother of Julia, age 2½, and Olivia, age 6 months
New Jersey

Have a babymoon before the baby comes. Gather your close friends around you a few weeks before you are due. Or even better yet, a couple of days or a week after you are due. Tell them to bring food and wine, music and laughter. Sit in a circle with great music and tell jokes. Sing songs (very cheesy, but it sure makes you laugh). There is nothing like calling the women who love you to you when you are ripe with child. They are there to ease your fears, make you laugh and cry, talk about you and your baby, and, of course, feed you. There is nothing else like it in the world. I was 17 days overdue with Mallaigh and called my women to me.

Sarah, doula and mother of Hannick, age 3, Kettie, age 2, and Mallaigh, age 8 weeks
Minnesota

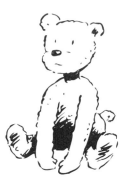

Decorating Nursery

Decorating a baby room is a wonderful opportunity to create a carefree hideaway – a place of slumber and lullabies. From Tropical Jungle to Noah's Ark, Teddy Bears to Winnie the Pooh: There are many delightful baby room themes to choose from – any one will spark enthusiasm and generate exciting nursery decorating ideas. But decorating the baby room can be daunting: There's so much choice – nursery bedding sets, furnishings, nursery wall décor, and accessories of all kinds! Coordinated nursery bedding sets and matching accessories can make easy work of decorating a baby room, ensuring nursery décor is effective and harmonious. But mixing and matching presents the opportunity for more imaginative nursery decorating ideas – and it's fun! The key to success with "mix and match" nursery décor is to select elements – baby nursery pictures, fabrics, and accessories – that share color and pattern elements. Basing nursery décor on neutral wall and floor coverings enables endless variations: Keeping baby room decorating ideas flexible makes it easy to adapt to a young child's developing interests. By changing just the accessories – nursery bedding sets, pictures, and rugs – different nursery decorating ideas can be developed without all the upheaval of a major redecorating project. For a while, at least, baby room themes can grow with your child!

Suzanne Brown, former special needs teacher and current writer and designer of teachers' educational materials and mother of Arthur, age 19
Penzance, UK

There are several nursery design considerations you need to take into account: color, furnishings, functionality, and convertibility are just a few of them. Color may be the single most important consideration when designing your baby's space. When babies are born, they can only see black and white. When they can see color, the first color they see is red. What this mean is that a room filled with soft blues may seem adorable to you, but it doesn't do anything for your child's early development. Additionally, studies show that babies cry more in yellow rooms, so a soft butter cream is also not the best choice at this stage. You may not be ready to paint the room a vibrant red, but consider a soft peach or neutral similar to the flesh color of the people who will spend the most time with your child. These colors will be associated with you and your family and will be soothing to the baby. Consider, also, creating contrast by using both dark and light shades of your colors. The contrast will help your child's ability to recognize shapes and objects.

Felicity Chapman, interior designer for Children's Spaces
California

There are so many ways to accessorize your new room. For wall decor you can take your favorite children's book to a local copy shop and ask them to color copy a few of the pictures. Simply framing the copies and hanging them on the wall with a wide ribbon will add a lovely addition to the decor. You can organize your changing table area with decorative lined baskets. Taking the linings to a local embroidery shop and asking them to embroider words such as Clothes, Diapers, and Necessities makes it easier for you to locate items. Boxes are a great way to keep small items, such as socks or photos, together. Purchase several paper mache boxes from your local craft store in different sizes and paint each one in a different color. Stacking these on top of each other, from large to small, will add a charming accent while providing the extra storage.

Amanda Dickson, owner/designer of PeaPod Creations, www.peapodcreations.com, and mother of Garret, age 6, and Michaela, age 2
Texas

Choose fabrics and rugs that are easy to clean. Avoid wall to wall carpeting. Instead, use area rugs which can be cleaned and/or replaced periodically. Instead of a framed picture, hang a quilt or fabric wall hanging near the crib – something that will not be dangerous if baby pulls it down.

Stacia Crawford, design consultant, owner of African Accents, and mother of Malcolm, age 5, Matthew, age 3, and Emmanuel, age 1
Illinois

Try something unexpected. Who says your nursery has to be baby blue or pink? I'm letting you "off the hook" from feeling committed to choosing a traditional nursery theme. Rather than a yellow ducky or storybook character theme, design a nursery in styles that you might have reflected throughout the rest of your home. Consider a French countryside theme with vivid colors, toile fabric, crystal chandelier, and a Louis XVI chair instead of a traditional rocking chair. Try an "old-world" Italian look with warm color-washed walls, a black iron crib, and warm terra cotta accents. An Asian-inspired room with silk fabric treatments in deep colors and sleek, dark wood furnishings with light colored walls would provide the bold contrast of colors that appeal to infants and parents alike. Many parents are opting for the vintage style in the nursery. These fabrics remind them of simpler times and their own childhoods. Soft, muted cotton print fabrics paired with vintage furniture will create a time tested and inviting atmosphere for all. Bright citrus colors are hot this year. Consider bright turquoise paired with orange or deep violet with sage green. These combinations would work for a baby girl or boy and are sure to turn some heads.

Most importantly, enjoy the process of preparing this nursery for your baby. This could very well be your only opportunity to have complete control over how this room looks. Decorate to please yourself. Think about it…the baby has no opinion on the room's colors or designs and won't even begin to care about the chosen theme or color scheme until he or she is at least three years old and, in most cases, even later. By this time, your little independent thinker will have his own ideas as to what he wants for his bedroom, and he will deserve to have the space reflect his own personality and interests.

Sherri Blum, C.I.D. (certified interior decorator), owner of Jack and Jill Interiors for Children and Bare Walls Design Co., and mother of Luke and Ethan
Maryland

Bed placement is important. Put the baby's bed on a solid wall across from the door with the head of the crib against the wall, rather than lengthwise, just as you would a regular bed. Too often parents put the long side of the crib against the wall instead of the head. Avoid doing this because the baby will be in a defensive position. After all, you wouldn't want to sleep with your bed against a wall, so don't place your baby that way. The bed should not be against a window or be directly in line with the door. Make sure the baby does not sleep or has a bed placed against a slanted wall or ceiling. These press on the baby. Avoid placing the baby against a wall that is shared with a bathroom, toilet, storage, or utility-type room.

Kathryn Weber, master Feng Shui consultant, publisher of *The Red Lotus Letter Feng Shui* e-zine (www.redlotusletter.com), and mother of Angela, age 14, and Steven, age 5
Texas

Choose versatile furniture to avoid having to purchase a new bed and dresser and sell a useless changing table in two years. Remember, this room will need to meet the needs of a rapidly changing and growing child with ever changing needs, interests, and attitudes. Most modern children's furniture is very versatile with cribs that convert to beds and dressers that double as changing tables. An armoire is another versatile option for a changing station. A contoured pad can be placed inside the doors. When no longer necessary, the pad can be removed; and the armoire can hold a television, computer, or hanging clothes. Don't purchase your typical primary colored plastic toy box. This will only suit for a few years. Instead, consider a wooden trunk that can later be used for sweater storage or a hope chest for a teenager. Convert a bookcase into toy storage by filling the shelves with fabric lined baskets to hold baby toys for now and then you have a bookcase to hold your growing child's book collection later.

Sherri Blum, C.I.D. (certified interior decorator), owner of Jack and Jill Interiors for Children and Bare Walls Design Co., and mother of Luke and Ethan
Maryland

Painting your nursery adds color and cheerfulness to the overall design. Choosing two or even three colors to paint with gives you many options that allow you to create something eye-catching. Using painter's tape, you can apply three colors to add horizontal stripes that blend up the wall. Apply one color for the bottom of the wall, another color for the center, and your third color for the top. Another idea to achieving a custom wall mural look is to paint all of the walls in a solid color and then hand paint a border around the top of the wall, using a secondary color to write phrases from a nursery rhyme. Phrases such as "Jack and Jill went up the hill…" and "Silver bells and cockle shells…" gives a nursery a fun and whimsical look while adding to the comfort of your room. You can purchase templates from your local craft store or by ordering online to create a more professional look.

Amanda Dickson, owner/designer of PeaPod Creations, www.peapodcreations.com, and mother of Garret, age 6, and Michaela, age 2
Texas

Unless you're going to love it for the next two to three years, I suggest you make the room warm and comfortable but not so "cutesy!" I have found that after one year, I'm so ready for a change to fit my baby's personality!

Dawn, domestic engineer and mother of
Miranda, age 11, Vinnie, age 7, and Alicia and Chad, age 4
Ohio

For the nursery or playroom choose artwork and accessories that touch you personally. It doesn't need to be childish, just interesting and well placed. Why not have a Van Gogh or Monet in your nursery? Babies love to look at faces and can see contrast easily, so consider framing an enlarged black and white photo of mom and dad or siblings. To make these even more interesting, use some heirloom or vintage fabrics from your own childhood as matting for these photos. Use your childhood train or doll collection as a display on shelving. This can be later built upon by your own child or replaced as time goes on with your child's own collection of choice. Don't neglect the ceiling. A baby spends most of his or her time on his/her back, looking at the ceiling. Make it interesting. A more realistic looking sky mural will last many years and will be calming for a child. The sky scene can reflect night or day or can fade from one into the other across the ceiling. At the very least, paint the ceiling some color other than white. Your child will thank you eventually!

Sherri Blum, C.I.D. (certified interior decorator), owner of Jack and Jill Interiors for Children and Bare Walls Design Co., and mother of Luke and Ethan
Maryland

Young children love bright primary colors but large areas can be overwhelming. Decorating the baby room with a subtle, calm color scheme is usually a better choice. Introducing warm colors – rose, peach, or primrose – into your baby room decorating ideas will help create a feeling of coziness. While decorating the baby room with the cool colors – aqua, mint, or sky blue – can create a feeling of spaciousness, it is probably best to keep ideas based on this color range for a room with a warm, sunny aspect. Touches of bright primary colors bring extra interest and visual stimulation. Introducing just small amounts with baby nursery pictures, nursery bedding sets, toys, and accessories can transform a room. These are the finishing touches that can bring nursery décor alive!

Suzanne Brown, former special needs teacher and current writer and designer of teachers' educational materials and mother of Arthur, age 19
Penzance, UK

Make an apple pie bed. That way the baby can't get lost under the sheets.

Michelle, play school teacher and mother of Matthew, age 7
England

Getting ready for a new baby requires a lot of thought and planning about everything from what diapers the baby will wear down to the decoration and arrangement of baby's room. Today's parents want to create a haven for their little one that will help their baby feel comforted and nurtured, as well as stimulated enough so that baby thrives. Increasingly, parents are going beyond the traditional coordinated "theme" rooms and incorporating feng shui to ensure baby not only has an attractive, but also harmonious, environment.

Feng shui, the Chinese system for arrangement and placement so often used in businesses and homes, is now making its way into the nursery, and for good reason, too. Feng shui proposes that by arranging and aligning the room correctly, energy will flow better in the room and that all who reside in the room will flourish and prosper better than if the energy in the room was not harmonious. Understandably, no one needs to thrive and flourish more than a baby.

To maximize the energy in baby's room, there are several important factors to consider, such as room location, safety, colors, and furniture arrangement. These make up the foundation of good feng shui in the nursery. Plus, using feng shui will help to make babies less fussy, make them feel more comfortable in their surroundings, and will promote their health and well-being. By following some of the most basic considerations, feng shui can help parents create a room that makes them AND their baby happy.

Kathryn Weber, master Feng Shui consultant, publisher of *The Red Lotus Letter Feng Shui* **e-zine (www.redlotusletter.com), and mother of Angela, age 14, and Steven, age 5**
Texas

I sandwich Kiley's sheets — one protective pad, one sheet, another pad, another sheet, and so on, usually four layers — so I can do a quick change (especially if she gets sick or dirty).

Tara, high school teacher and at-home-mother of Kiley, age 2
California

I have a changing table that is a difficult shape to fit a cover on, and I do not want to spend the money on the covers for it. We have an abundance of crib sheets, though, so what I do is use a fitted crib sheet instead of a changing table pad, and then place a small changing pad on top to protect the sheet. I simply tuck the sheet under; and if I am worried about it coming loose, then I simply pin the two sides together underneath.

Amy Clark, owner/founder of www.momadvice.com, and mother of Ethan, age 2
Indiana

One of the most exciting things to do when you are expecting is to design and decorate the nursery for your new arrival. Your nursery can look as though you hired a professional without paying the high prices. Fabric is the key design when decorating and is the main focal point in the room. Decide on a color scheme, style, and overall feel that will bring comfort to you and your baby. There are many choices when it comes to fabric so don't feel overwhelmed. Simply choose your fabrics one at a time, adding as many as you would like. An affordable way to choose fabric for your crib bedding is to purchase large sheets and linens. These fabrics are usually affordable with a high thread count and an array of styles. Two large king-size sheets can be made into a bumper, skirt, sheet, blanket, and even window treatments. With several crib bedding patterns from your local fabric shop, you can have a friend or relative sew your bedding while adding a sentimental value to the nursery. If you don't know anyone who sews, many custom crib bedding stores will allow you to supply your own fabric with you only having to pay for their service.

Amanda Dickson, owner/designer of PeaPod Creations, www.peapodcreations.com, and mother of Garret, age 6, and Michaela, age 2
Texas

Two essential items: a light with a dimmer switch and black-out curtains.

Jenny
California

From a series of framed art prints to big cheerful posters, a collage of birthday cards to giant stick-ups – nursery wall décor can create an interesting focus and highlight of color. A special picture may provide inspiration for some great baby nursery ideas and the basis for a subtle color scheme. Pictures can be used to develop baby room themes, giving them added dimension: Baby nursery pictures of animals can extend a tropical jungle theme; Paddington Bear pictures, a teddy bear theme. Look for baby nursery pictures that you find inspiring – they can be a valuable source for interesting nursery decorating ideas. But, best of all, good nursery wall décor will help to create a special place that excites whimsical fantasy and imaginative storytelling – the essence of a magical childhood!

Suzanne Brown, former special needs teacher and current writer and designer of teachers' educational materials and mother of Arthur, age 19
Penzance, UK

Choose a theme for your nursery but make sure it's versatile and can grow with your child so it can last several years. Choose wall treatments and furniture that are versatile and save the babyish feeling accessories for smaller items that can be changed easily. Make sure the nursery has a comfortable chair or rocker. You will be spending a lot of time there.

Stacia Crawford, design consultant, owner of African Accents, and mother of Malcolm, age 5, Matthew, age 3, and Emmanuel, age 1
Illinois

Here are tips for creating good feng shui in your baby's room:

1. Select a good location for the baby's bedroom.
A new baby should have a bedroom that is not over a garage or has an empty space below. The bedroom also shouldn't be located where there is excessive noise that might keep the baby from sleeping, such as close to a living room where the TV is on or close to a noisy street or neighbor.

2. Opt for soothing colors.
Children benefit from bright colors in play areas, but if these are used in a baby's room, infants can be over stimulated to the point that they do not rest well. Because deep sleep in babies is necessary for healthy growth, be sure to select restful, muted colors. Whites are excellent for children, but avoid a black and white color scheme because there is too much contrast. Select color palettes that are close to one another and harmonious in feng shui terms, such as green and blue, white and beige, or pink and yellow.

3. Create soft movement in the room.
A room that is too still becomes stagnant, and this is not beneficial for the growth of the child. To create good, but soft energy and movement, hang mobiles close to a window to move gently in the breeze and keep soft music playing in the room. You can also place a small fan on a dresser turned on low to keep air moving in the room. Avoid placing the baby under a ceiling fan as these disrupt their body energy.

4. Watch for pointed objects.
Make sure there are no hard corners from dressers or changing tables pointed at the baby's head or body. Move these to another part of the room where they are not pointed in the direction of the bed.

Kathryn Weber, master Feng Shui consultant, publisher of *The Red Lotus Letter Feng Shui* e-zine (www.redlotusletter.com), and mother of Angela, age 14, and Steven, age 5
Texas

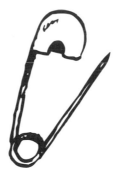

Baby Care Stations

Set up a changing station on each floor of the house. Have diapers, wipes, extra outfits, and blankets at each one. Put a cotton ball and Q-tip holder and a bottle of isopropyl alcohol on baby's changing table(s) for cleaning the umbilical cord. The alcohol squares they send you home from the hospital with really don't clean down in the crevices like a Q-tip can. Newborn boys have a nasty habit of squirting <u>everything</u> when you change their diaper. Have a breast pad or washcloth on the changing table and put it on them <u>as soon as you remove the dirty diaper</u>. (Don't worry, this gets better after the first month!)

Get several waterproof cotton changing pads, large and small. Have plenty of newborn gowns ("sacs") or terry pajamas. Expect to use 3 to 4 <u>a day</u> at first! Get 6 to 12 "pre-folded" cloth diapers for burp cloths and under baby's head in the crib or your bed. Get a small dishpan and keep it on the washer for soaking soiled baby clothes (and underwear).

Brooke A. Schumacher, M.D., and mother of a daughter, age 3, and twin sons, age 1½
Dhahran, Saudi Arabia

Make yourself a little breastfeeding basket that you can take with you from room to room. Some good things to include are diapers, wipes, burp clothes, extra baby clothes, a book or magazine, the phone, the remote control, some energy bars, a baby toy, etc.

Stacey, anthropologist and mother of
Satchel, age 2, and Jiro, age 5 months
Tennessee

I sewed pockets onto my Boppy to keep a water bottle and spit cloth.

Dolores, R.N., Lamaze(LCCE), doula, and mother of Jonathon and Megan
New York

I made "nursing stations" all over my house. I just got small baskets and filled them with diapers, wipes, burp clothes, diaper rash ointment, books to entertain other children, snacks, and water bottles. I put one in each room I would nurse in (in front of the TV, beside my bed, etc.) so that everything was always easily accessible, and I could just sit down and feed my baby wherever I was. It saved so much time over keeping everything in the baby's room or on a changing table.

Tania, labor doula and childbirth educator (CAPPA) and mother of
Stephen, age 13, Brendan, age 11, Kathryn, age 9, and Michael, age 7
Colorado

I set up a changing station in our kitchen. I simply cleared out a cabinet above the counter and filled it with diapers, clothing, towels, blankets, bottles, ointments, etc. I put a changing pad on the counter underneath the cabinet. I taped a black and white photo above the pad, so while I was changing my son he could look up at it and be amused. It saved me sooo many trips going up the stairs. I thought it was ingenious!

Monique, mother of Hunter, age 4, and Tanner, age 17 months
California

Have a nursing station set up in each area of the house where you plan to feed the baby. Don't forget to include:

1. a case of bottled water — drink, drink, drink while baby is feeding

2. breast pads — in case both breasts let down at the same time; also to protect your clothes against lanolin nipple ointment

3. a clock that you can read in the dark and a soothing CD and player

4. several kinds of pacifiers to see which kind baby might like (Babies need to suck, and orthodontists say pacifiers are better than a thumb.)

5. pen and paper to keep track of feeding times and duration, breast used, etc. (It really does help to do this when you first begin since you are tired, sore, befuddled, and newly in love!)

The contributing moms of "The List," a growing list of
new mom tips passed from friend to friend
New Jersey, Maryland, and Delaware

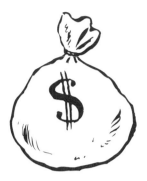

Financial Planning

Buy one package of diapers and wipes with each paycheck. Buying necessities ahead of time will help save money after baby arrives. If you're planning on staying home after your baby arrives, start living on one paycheck as soon as possible. The amount you save will act as a nice cushion for unexpected expenses or a good start for baby's college fund.

**Kim Danger, owner www.mommysavers.com, and mother of
Sydney, age 5, and Nicholas, age 1
Minnesota**

This is the time to investigate life insurance and draw up wills. Taking care of these things now will reduce stress later.

**Abigail, mortgage broker and mother of Karen, age 3, and Kyle, age 4 months
Washington, D.C.**

If you both work and one of you plans to stay home with the baby, you should immediately begin to live off your one income and put the other aside. This will help you become acclimated to your new financial situation long before the baby comes so that on top of the stress of a newborn, you aren't faced with a different household budget.

**Kathi, mother of Matthew, age 6, Allison, age 4, and Miranda, age 8 months
Alabama**

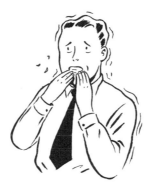

— Preparing Your Partner —

Prepare yourself, your partner, and your family and friends by setting up a support system that allows you to be with your baby as much as possible for the first year. Tell everyone how important they will be to you in your new motherhood. Ask them to commit to bringing you food; running errands; doing laundry; doing dishes; vacuuming; being with baby for short whiles so that you can take a long bath or eat a relaxing meal in front of the TV; rubbing your back and feet, etc. (so that you can do the same for your husband). ANYTHING that will make it easier for you to respond to your baby in the way that your heart will want you to will be good. It is not possible to do too much for a new mom.

**Meladee, courtesy of The Center for Conscious Parenting, www.cfcp.info, teacher who is currently a very happy stay-at-home mother of Colin, age 5½, and Rory, age 11 months
Oregon**

My husband will always tell new dads-to-be that the amount of sacrifice they make will help them tremendously with bonding. By that he means getting up in the night, helping mother to nurse, being supportive, looking after baby as well as bathing, settling, and holding. Fathers who do this get to know baby and to understand better what a hard job it is for mum.

**Adith, La Leche League leader studying to be a childbirth educator, and mum of Eden and Finn
Auckland, New Zealand**

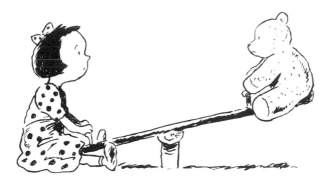

— Preparing Your Kids —

To have an open, honest relationship with your older child before the baby comes doesn't mean saying things to make him/her feel good. When parents tell their child that they love him so much they have decided to have another one to love, it is no more comforting to that child than your husband telling you he loves you so much that he's going to get a new wife, and "we'll all be one big happy family." Your child is highly dependent on you for a relationship that includes honesty, security, nurturing, and patience. After that relationship is established, you can implement some practical things to prepare your child for the new baby. I see that when my youngest children have play babies, they play with them in nurturing ways. "Be gentle with a baby" is a common saying around my house. "We're supposed to protect the baby" is another way to encourage respect once you already have a good relationship. I typically show my little ones a picture of a pregnant mom in a book such as *What to Expect When You're Expecting*. I like the five, six, and seven mother pictures that show the baby upside down in Mommy's tummy. By then, they can identify the shape of your tummy with the picture, and it helps to visualize the "precious cargo" you're carrying. I let them feel the baby move, and I let them "hug" the baby and tell him/her "goodnight."

Susan, mother of Rebecca, age 17, Catherine, age 15, Philip, age 12, Paul, age 11, Marybeth, age 9, Hannah, age 8, Matthew, age 6, Mark, age 4, Joshua, age 3, and Joann, age 11 months
Texas

When I was pregnant, I prepared the older sibling by telling him that "Mommy will be holding the baby and nursing the baby all the time." I've told him that we can still do things together while the baby nurses or is in the sling. This way the older sibling doesn't feel that the baby is getting in the way of his relationship with his mommy.

Amy, mother of Oliver, age 8, Sam, age 5, Owen, age 2, and Milo, 2 weeks
Georgia

If you have another child at home, pack a day/overnight bag for him/her and keep it ready, just in case you need to make a quick "drop off" on the way to the hospital. Include some favorite books, toys, and a picture of Mommy and Daddy, as well as clothes, pajamas, and diapers or underwear. Prepare a list of emergency phone numbers and any instructions for the sitter and keep it with the packed bag.

Brooke A. Schumacher, M.D., and mother of a daughter, age 3, and twin sons, age 1½
Dhahran, Saudi Arabia

What seemed to work for my daughter was talking about the fact that she was going to be a big sister. We watched some videos and read a lot of books about babies and what it is to be a big sister. This, we think, seemed to ease the transition of a baby coming into her life. We also tried to keep her same schedule of activities without much interruption. A combination of things like these helped introduce her little brother and be as accepting as a 2-year-old can be.

Sol Cristina, mother of Isabel Paloma, age 3, and David Sebastian, age 8 months
California

When I was pregnant with my second son, I didn't realize how much of an impact it would have on my first son. When the baby was born, Donovan (the oldest) was turning 2 in two days. When he came to see the baby and me at the hospital, he told his dad and me to put the baby back. He wanted nothing to do with a new baby. When I was pregnant with my third son, I included both of the older children in doctors visits and talks about the new baby. Donovan was now 4½ and my second son, Shane, was 2½. When the baby was born, both children wanted to help with the care of the baby. Learning from this, I wish I had included Donovan in the process the first time. I feel it's important to include all of the children, even if you're having your second, third, fourth, etc. Make the bond between you and your children strong. My sons are still very close to me, and they are 17, 15, and 12.

Michele, owner of a home business and mother of
Donovan, age 17, Shane, age 15, and Travis, age 12
Colorado

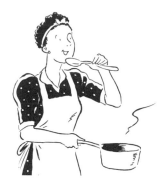

Preparing Yourself

After having a baby, you may feel too fatigued to cook when you return from the hospital, so cook, label, and freeze meals in single portions before you go. Defrost and reheat them as desired.

**Amy Clark, owner/founder of www.momadvice.com, and mother of Ethan, age 2
Indiana**

Make a labor project list and a meal angels list. Include 10 things you might do in early/pre-labor. Examples are: pack the bag, take a walk outside, bake cookies (you'll know it's time to go to your birthplace when the cookies start to burn!). For the meal angels, assign 10 people you know who could bring you meals after the baby comes. Include their contact information and give the list to a trusted helper and have them contact and organize two weeks worth of great meals!

**Jesse, childbirth educator, birth doula, and mother of Dashiell, age 1
Oregon**

Pre-prepare healthy meals in advance and freeze them so that when you are tired with a newborn or alone, you will have a good meal to eat.

**Judith, self-employed and mother of Miranda, age 8, Jadeen, age 6,
Erin, age 3, and Mercedes, age 8 months
Queensland, Australia**

During the last few weeks of pregnancy, make up meals and freeze them so you don't have to cook when baby arrives!

Stacey, nanny and mother of Matthew, age 5 months
London, England

Get a good pump, a nursing bra, and read a book on breastfeeding BEFORE you have your baby. Try to get a breastfeeding buddy – someone who has recently breastfed and can offer you support if you have any problems. Breastfeeding is an art, but it needs to be learned like anything else, so don't give up if it is difficult in the beginning. It will get better!

Stacey, anthropologist and mother of Satchel, age 2, and Jiro, age 5 months
Tennessee

As fellow women who have recently gone through this ourselves, we want to share what we have learned. Here's what you should have waiting for you after the baby arrives.

1. a large box of Always extra, extra, extra absorbent pads (You may bleed up to a month after delivery.)

2. comfy maternity underwear, pants, and shirts — just comfy anything!

3. Ibuprofen — helps with episiotomies and breastfeeding pain

4. beer — one beer before breastfeeding can help with let-down reflex

5. Soothies gel pads (available in the baby/nursing section of the drug store) for very sore nipples

The contributing moms of "The List," a growing list of
new mom tips passed from friend to friend
New Jersey, Maryland, and Delaware

Attend moms groups, La Leche League, or other playgroups BEFORE your baby arrives so that you have a support group in place when you need them, and you know that you are not alone.

Marisa, mother of Elijah, age 2½, and Marin, age 9 months
California

Remember, your body is changing. Your body is beautiful, strong, and powerful!

Jennifer, certified childbirth educator and mother of Amanda, age 5½, and Abby,
age 2½
Georgia

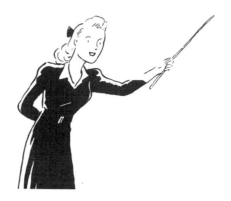

Prenatal Classes

Childbirth classes are an excellent idea for first-time parents. All the reading in the world does not prepare you or your significant other for actual childbirth.

Dawn, RN, and mother of Sophia, age 3, and Analiese, age 1
New Jersey

I learned hypnosis for childbirth and had a very positive birth experience. I can not imagine labour without this positive tool. I would encourage anyone who is pregnant to at least look into this as a means of educating yourself to prepare for childbirth. It took away the stress and made me in control of my body for the best shot at a natural birth.

Leslie, mother of Connor William, age 16 months
Ontario, Canada

If you are planning to try natural birth (no medication), take a Bradley Method class and definitely prepare and practice alternative positions for giving birth other than just lying on your back. You will have a better chance at not tearing or needing an episiotomy.

Andrea, desktop support specialist and mother of
Leah Athena, age 1 month
New Jersey

Make sure you feel relaxed and good about yourself and the birth when you leave class. A good childbirth class should not be scary!

Ilana Stein, doula trainer and mentor and childbirth educator
New York

Prepare for your birth! You can have a beautiful birth experience. Learn as much as you can about the labor and delivery process. Read and take childbirth education classes. Knowledge reduces the fear of the unknown factor. Introspect: be honest about your needs for the optimum birth experience. Hire labor support to help realize your vision. Finally, make sure that you and your birth team are all working together.

Monet, doula, Lamaze childbirth educator, and mother of
Yisroel, age 6, Shayna, age 4, and Ari, age 2
New York

Start attending La Leche League while you're still pregnant. Breastfeeding is natural, but you still have to learn how to do it. Knowledge is power! The more you learn about breastfeeding BEFORE you have to do it, the easier it will be! LLL LOVES having pregnant women at their meetings, and it's a great way to watch other breastfeeding women to get used to seeing exactly how it's done.

Sarah, stay-at-home mother of
Adam, age 3, and Baby #2 due February 2005
Oklahoma

Prepare yourself to breastfeed by finding the best and most empathetic lactation expert available — one who has breastfed her own children and who will not let you give up when the going gets tough. Find other expectant mothers and experienced mothers with the same goals through LLL, Attachment Parenting International, or your church. (It helps to know a mom with at least one child who is 10 months to 2 years old as older moms sometimes forget what the challenges were like.) Get phone numbers and call these women when you have questions.

Meladee, courtesy of The Center for Conscious Parenting, www.cfcp.info, teacher
who is currently a very happy stay-at-home mother of Colin, age 5½,
and Rory, age 11 months
Oregon

Attend a La Leche League meeting or other breastfeeding support groups before your baby is born. Plan to breastfeed for at least six weeks. Those first weeks are the hardest, but afterward it does get easier. And keep that La Leche League leader's phone number easily accessible from your nursing area in case you do have trouble!

Mara, La Leche League leader, counselor when employed, and stay-at-home mother of Gabrielle, age 4, and Alexander, age 1
Georgia

Before you deliver, take a breastfeeding class and make a resources list of breastfeeding advocates. Make sure your pediatrician is a breastfeeding advocate. Most say they are, but are they really? How they deal with jaundice is a great issue to really figure out. Research has shown that breastfeeding helps eliminate bilirubin from your baby's system better than sugar water or formula substitutes. Therefore, why would any doctor advise a mother to STOP breastfeeding when her baby is jaundice (which occurs in about half of all infants) when breastfeeding has shown to be better? Too bad I didn't have this research and information for my first baby. Switching her from breast to sugar water during her first days was a nightmare for my body as well as hers. She never did latch on well, and I, consequently, gave up. I needed more professional support. And, yes, she did have multiple ear infections which sent me to the doctor's office every two weeks for the first five years of her life. Eventually, she had ear surgery for tube replacement. When I stand back and look at the circumstances and events, I wish I had asked for the "research." At least I would have had the opportunity to make a better choice. When it comes to moms, they really do know best. Medical advice is still advice, and a medical guess is still nothing more than an educated guess. Trust in yourself; if it doesn't feel right – don't do it until you have the information you need.

JaLynn, mother of Kassie, age 14, and Kayla, age 7
Michigan

For some breastfeeding comes easily; for others, not so easy. Breastfeeding is a learned art. It takes practice, patience, and perseverance. Before baby is born, make sure you have a support system established (i.e., La Leche League), know where to get help should you have trouble (lactation consultant), read all you can about breastfeeding, and, if possible, attend a breastfeeding class. Tell yourself you will breastfeed, not that you will "try." Positive affirmations work!

Yvonne, birth and postpartum doula and mother of Jordan, age 13, Jacob, age 10, Jared, age 8, Jacy, age 7, Joshua, age 5, Jianna, age 4, and Jessica, age 2.
Colorado

We all think that breastfeeding should be a natural instinctive thing to do. I think the most surprising part is that it isn't always easy, that it takes time, and unless you are committed, most likely you will not succeed. I have nursed four children for various lengths of time – from eight months to over two-and-a-half years. At times it was frustrating, difficult, and even painful; but the rewards were well worth the time, effort, and patience. The thing that surprised me the most was that my previous experience never helped me with subsequent children. Just as different as they look and act, they start out different from the moment they latch on! I suggest finding a resource of mothers, such as the La Leche League, to assist you. It is best to go to the meetings before your baby arrives so that you have a relationship with the person you may need to call in case a need arises. Although your hospital may have lactation consultants, I have noticed in my doula practice that moms who choose to find support in La Leche League often have the best results. The relationship with other moms going through or getting through various experiences seems to really be a benefit.

**Michelle, LMT, CD, apprenticing midwife and mother of
Josh, age 13, Hannah, age 9, Hailey, age 6, and Johnathon Hunter, age 3
Utah**

Breastfeeding was one of the highlights and proud accomplishments of my daughter's first year. My recommendation is to prepare as much as possible in advance. I read *The Nursing Mother's Companion* cover to cover, observed another mom nursing, and attended a breastfeeding class all before my daughter's birth. I knew that it might be difficult and not come naturally. The preparation paid off. I developed an infection that came very close to ending our nursing relationship before it even started. Without my preparation, education, and resources, I would only have breastfed a few days. I attended a weekly breastfeeding education and support group at the hospital where I birthed. After seeing several lactation consultants, renting a hospital grade pump for one month, and holding on through the pain and the occasional tears, I fully enjoyed nursing my daughter through the end of her first year. It was truly an investment in her health and development as well as the closeness of our relationship. Be prepared, get education, and ask for help!

**Kate, counselor and mother of Isabella, age 17 months
New Jersey**

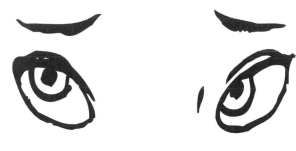

Fears & Anxiety

Birth doesn't have to be painful, especially when a mother is completely free from fear. We are all mammals, and we should remember that our bodies will respond like other mammals by shutting down the birthing process when it is removed from a comfortable environment. Consider having your baby at home with a qualified home midwife, a statistically safer place to give birth for healthy mothers. If you feel that you must go to a hospital, stay home as long as possible to reduce your odds for interventions. Interventions can easily snowball in birth, often with one leading to many within hours. We know that nearly all female mammals have bodies perfectly designed to give birth. It is the interventions which interfere with the process, and that begins with the first intervention that occurs when a mother leaves home to give birth elsewhere. We live in a highly medically managed society where many mothers have birth done to them and not with them. It is no wonder that almost one in three moms end up having their babies surgically removed from their bodies. Do not allow yourself to believe that birth is an emergency waiting to happen. Millions of years of evolution have brought us here, and so we can not assume that birth has become dangerous all of a sudden. No mother deserves to have a new baby and major abdominal surgery at the same time. There is so much that you can do to keep you and your baby safe, and you might be surprised to learn that going to the hospital is, for most moms, on the very bottom of that list. Birth truly is as safe as life gets.

Kelley, childbirth educator and mother of Simon, age 2
Massachusetts

Don't let anyone scare you about labor and delivery. People make it worse than it truly is. I had an amazing experience, and I can't wait to be pregnant again.

Fanya, mother of Sasha, age 8 months
California

I cannot stress enough how important it is that you NOT watch television shows featuring real-life births and that you NOT listen to every birthing story being replayed by proud mothers. Television tends to show very dramatic births rather than the calm, beautiful experience that it can be. Your birth will not be like any other you have seen or heard of because it is yours. You will have a much nicer birth if you load up on positive, confidence building thoughts throughout your pregnancy.

Kathleen, homemaker and mother of Mary Elizabeth, age 6 months
New Mexico

Try very hard not to listen to others' "war stories" before giving birth. Each experience is as unique and wonderful as the child you've created.

Amy, stay-at-home mother of Weston, age 3½, Hank, age 13 months,
and 6 months pregnant
Illinois

Look forward to your labor! You don't have to be afraid of it. It's an amazing, never to be replicated experience that you and your baby will share as you work together towards birth.

Kristin, mother of Conor, age 5 and born in a hospital, and
Bella, age 7 months and born at home in the water
Washington

Surround yourself with people who have had positive birth experiences! Since so many people are willing to share "their story," make sure they are ones that are positive and encouraging, not scary or disheartening. Birth will be a beautiful and easier experience if you have heard that it can be from other women.

Brandy, professional birth assistant and mother of a little boy, age 7 months
Colorado

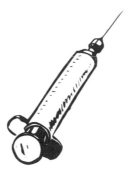

The Pediatrician

Set up three "interviews" to find that perfect person! You should get that "I love this person" feeling. You'll know it's the right decision! After all, this person will be seeing a lot of your child.

**Dawn, domestic engineer and mother of
Miranda, age 11, Vinnie, age 7, and Alicia and Chad, age 4
Ohio**

Become an advocate for your child, even before he/she is born! Learn all you can by reading books, searching the internet, and asking your doctor questions. Don't just accept the first, or even second, opinion. Be knowledgeable so that you can make the most informed decision for your child.

**Julie, purchasing manager, Chinaberry Inc., www.chinaberry.com,
and mother of two
California**

Seek a doctor of chiropractic who can provide prenatal and pediatric care for you and your little one. It makes a world of difference for a healthy pregnancy, birth, and child. Find a dedicated and caring doctor at www.ICPA4kids.com.

**Colleen Holland, doctor of chiropractic and mother of Amelia, age 9 months
Colorado**

Keep in mind that most doctors have a little bit of basic knowledge about a lot of topics. If you are told something that doesn't sound right, don't just assume that the doctor knows best – he may not. Another doctor may have more (or less) information on the subject and will tell you something completely different. Use any available resource to find out more and then make an educated decision based on your findings. Don't be afraid to trust your instincts.

Beth Foster, certified lactation consultant, consultant for Natural Family Boutique, and mother of Nicholas, age 5, Alexander, age 3, and Baby #3 due in March '05. Kentucky

I know this seems obvious, but remember that your child's pediatrician is a specialist hired by you; and if you are not comfortable, find another! Know your child's body and how it responds to illness. My son, who is now 18, has a low body temperature of 97.1, which means when his temperature reaches 99, he's sick! He also had strep throat infections with little or no redness or sore throat. If you recognize your child is ill and take him to the pediatrician, insist on tests that he/she would otherwise not offer to do, just because your child does not appear ill to him/her! I once insisted on a quick strep test in the doctor's office, which the pediatrician reluctantly did, and my son had a raging step infection! Trust your feelings when your child is ill!

Karen, insurance compliance and mother of Colin Jeremy, age 18 New Jersey

Keeping young children entertained during all of those doctor visits can be a real challenge. Bring along a gallon-size zipper lock bag and a dry-erase marker. Your little ones can slip a magazine into the bag and draw, trace, and doodle through the plastic. Erase with a tissue and start again.

Deborah Shelton, author of *The Five Minute Parent: Fun & Fast Activities for You and Your Little Ones* and mother of Kizer, age 6

Your doctor is an expert on medical issues, which is a good thing if you need medical advice. But he or she is probably not an expert on breastfeeding, nutrition, sleep issues, etc. If your doctor offers advice in these areas, you don't need to feel guilty about ignoring it. If you need advice in these areas, consult a La Leche League leader, a nutritionist, or whoever has the education and expertise needed to answer your questions.

Beverly, editor and mother of Julia, age 24, and Eric, age 18 New Jersey

Read up on signs and symptoms of dehydration. Know what to do. Realize when you need to get the child to a hospital, even if the doctor doesn't think it's necessary. I took my daughter to the pediatrician's office in the morning, after days of vomiting and diarrhea many times, overnight as well. She hadn't peed since 8 pm the night before and still didn't until 11 am. When she did, it was dark brown. She was lethargic even at the office. Her skin wasn't as bad as they thought it should be if she was dehydrated, so they told me to continue trying to give her fluids and a BRAT diet (bananas, rice, applesauce, and toast). She continued to throw up. She became more lethargic. I finally just took her to the hospital.

She was so dehydrated that they admitted her for the entire weekend. The pediatrician told them that she didn't "look" that bad. Her blood showed she was dangerously dehydrated. So, trust your maternal instincts. If you instinctively feel that something is wrong with your child, push to have the child see a specialist for peace of mind. The doctors only see your child for a short visit. You know what your child has been doing, how he/she has been feeling, and what has been happening over the long-term. Keep notes of anything you feel is important. Make a list of what to ask the doctor, if necessary, because they won't always know something is wrong unless you tell them.

Debbie, owner of www.coconutbeach.com, and mother of
CJ, age 6½, and Rachel, age 2
New Jersey

Make sure that the pediatrician you select is not only someone you trust to care for your baby, but someone you feel comfortable with as well. There will be many times in the first year when you call the office. Make sure they do not make you feel bad or silly for calling. A large part of being a good pediatrician is handling nervous parents.

Jane, mother of Nicholas, age 3, and Sam and Will, age 16 months
New Jersey

Try and attend a short first aid homeopathy course with other new mums. It gives you some control and saves running to the doctor, anxious about your children.

Catherine, nurse, nursery proprietor, and mother of
Sinead, age 8, Ciara, age 5, Rosin, age 4, and Sean, age 1
W. Yorks, United Kingdom

Always trust your instincts when it comes to your child's health. Don't be afraid to seek "alternative" answers for health issues. My son went through an awful time with earaches and headaches at the age of 2. After trying all of the traditional methods with no lasting relief, we found an answer with craniosacral therapy and nutritional support. He was earache and headache free almost immediately and has had no reoccurrences. Best of all, he actually enjoyed the therapy!

Elaine, bookkeeper and mother of Jeffrey, age 5
Massachusetts

I would like to say that if you really feel strongly that your child is not well, follow it up with your doctor. My son was diagnosed with liver cancer at 13 months. This only happened because I refused to go home from the doctor's office until he sent me, albeit very reluctantly, directly to the local hospital. I subsequently found out my son had been very close to death. I don't blame the doctor, as my son's condition was very rare, but things hadn't been right for a long time, and I kept being fobbed off. Silly things occurred, like his nails weren't strong; he cried and cried when he was put in the bouncer; he couldn't digest lumpy food. There were many more symptoms which individually don't seem odd, but collectively summated to something not quite right. We were lucky that after immediate medical intervention and many months of agonizing ups and downs, he is now a healthy 9-year-old. So I repeat…follow your feelings as you know your child best.

Jane, child care worker
England

Insist that your pediatrician perform one of the developmental tests recommended by the American Academy of Pediatrics: The PEDS, the Child Development Inquiry, or The Ages and Stages Questionnaires. These tests only take minutes and are far more accurate then just asking a few questions and observing your child in the office. The earlier delays are discovered, the earlier you can get therapies, and the more effective those therapies will be.

Nancy, writer and mother of Dante, age 5
New York

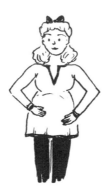

Feeling Uncomfortable

I found that a great way to keep cool and get relief from swollen feet was to wrap my feet in wet towels. It made me much cooler without freezing the rest of the family, and it relieved the swelling in my feet.

Lashawn, stay-at-home mother of James, age 9, Justin, age 5, Mackenzie, age 2, and Miles, age 2 months
Florida

★

Don't worry when your feet look like they're about to burst out of your shoes. Stay positive and be sure to check with your doctor that there isn't too much swelling. Swollen ankles won't last forever. But do make sure that after you've had your baby, you get a lot of rest and relaxation as well as begin some form of exercise. Swollen ankles are forgivable when you're pregnant; but when you don't have a bun in the oven, they're just plain unsightly…most of all to you.

Jennifer
North Carolina

I have been experiencing discomfort in the pubic area for about the past two or three weeks. After receiving the Prenatal Cradle, I wore it all day at work, and it helped with the discomfort immensely. I am also an avid exerciser and still do uphill treadmill walks almost everyday, and the support I receive from the cradle is fantastic. It has made a huge difference for me. It's also very discreet and comfortable to wear.

Jennifer K.
Ohio

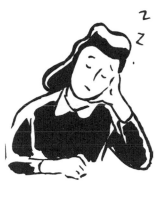

So Tired

While pregnant, make sure you go to bed on a regular schedule and don't stay up late. I took the advice from a friend, and I have never had a problem putting my 22-month-old to bed.

Leslie, teacher and mother of Rylee, age 22 months
Texas

Sleep is not cumulative. No matter how much you sleep during your pregnancy, especially near the end, you will still be exhausted after the baby is born!

Jessica H.

Sleep now, no matter how uncomfortable you may feel, especially toward the end of your term. You will still be getting a more consistent opportunity to sleep at the end of your pregnancy than you will the first three months of your baby's life!

Catherine, business owner and mother of Dylan, age 16, and Will, age 13
Colorado

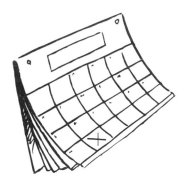

The Last Month

Avoid reclining during the last few weeks of your pregnancy. Doing so will help prevent painful back labor.

**Kelly, doula, childbirth educator, and stay-at-home mother of
Siri, age 8, Gunnar, age 6, Annaliese, age 3, and Sven, age 3
Washington**

During your last few weeks of pregnancy, remember to enjoy the pleasures of life without a baby. Soon it's going to take lots of planning to be able to go out to dinner and lots of luck to have uninterrupted sex!

**Sheryl Gurrentz, author of *The Guilt-Free Guide to Your New Life as a Mom* and
If Your Child is Bipolar and mother of Jordan, age 13, and Joey, age 10
Colorado**

If your baby is breech, take some time out to really relax. Talk to your baby and reassure him/her that all is well, that you are looking forward to welcoming him/her into the world, and he/she is loved and wanted. Tell him/her that the birth will be easier if he/she is head down. Look at a picture of a baby in the best position for birth and imagine your baby moving into that position.

**Moira Campbell, HypnoBirthing practitioner and mother of
Calum, age 5, and Isobel, age 2
British Columbia, Canada**

Order/buy announcements and get the envelopes addressed before the baby comes. Have your return address printed on them or use address stickers. Have plenty of thank-you notes and stamps in the house. At 37 weeks, wash <u>everything</u> you have for the baby: clothes, blankets, sheets, etc. Wash toys in hot soapy water or dishwasher, if possible. Get a good supply of film and camera batteries. Also, charge up the video camera batteries.

Buy several nursing pajamas (or 2-piece pajamas with a short top) that you really like and plan to spend the first two weeks postpartum in them. Get plenty of breast pads: Pigeon brand disposable breast pads are the best. They are individually wrapped, have adhesive, and are really absorbent! I would have 3 to 4 boxes of 24 in the house before the baby is born.

Put a basket on the back of each toilet stocked with sanitary pads (at first, the most absorbent and longest you can buy), underwear, your squirt bottle from the hospital, and breast pads. Put a small trash can right next to each toilet. Take the squirt bottle home from the hospital and use it at least 3 to 6 times a day the first week. Use it in the shower. Get some cheap (or disposable) underwear that you can afford to get stained and then discard the first week or two. Or have a generous supply of your designated "old" underwear.

I hope you find these suggestions as helpful as I did. They came from many friends, patients, and my own experience. Whether this is your first baby or you already have children, you are about to experience a miracle. It is a stressful time, too, and I wish you all the best as you enjoy/endure it.

**Brooke A. Schumacher, M.D., and mother of a daughter, age 3, and twin sons, age 1½
Dhahran, Saudi Arabia**

Add two weeks to your due date. That is when you can "expect" the baby to come. And don't listen to the doctor who tells you that you are three centimeters dilated and 80% effaced and could go into labor at any moment.

**Jill, full-time mother of Alison, age 1
Illinois**

If you can, speak to your doctor about a sleep aid for the night early labor begins so that you can sleep in preparation for the hard work of active labor which lies ahead. I ask my moms to ask their physicians about Ambien which, I have been told, is safe for baby as well.

Taffy, doula

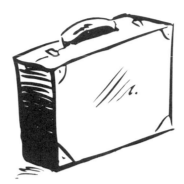

Bring to the Hospital

Being a birth doula, I have made a list of several things over the years moms have wished for once at the hospital:

1. Your own soft toilet paper.

2. A calling card for long distance calls.

3. Your own pillows with dark cases, so not to get mixed up with hospital ones.

4. Snack-size bag of pretzels. After delivery at 3 in the morning, moms are famished; and while nurses are trying to locate a dinner tray for you, you can snack on pretzels.

5. Two pairs of socks for both you and your baby. Moms may get one pair wet, and often times baby's feet don't stay wrapped in the blankets.

6. Lip balm.

7. Baby book or a white T-shirt for dad to get baby's foot prints on when the hospital does them.

8. Several copies of the birth wish list. Sometimes at shift changes the wish list gets lost, so have a copy for everyone who is to take care of you.

9. An object to use as a focal point. Some moms choose baby's first teddy bear; others, pictures. This can be anything you can really concentrate on.

10. Change of clothes for dad.

11. Camera.

**Dawn, birth doula and mother of
Stephanie, age 19, Peter, age 17, Craig, age 10, and Kimberly, age 8
Maryland**

Take your Bobby Pillow or Breast Friend pillow. It will be a back saver whether bottle feeding or breastfeeding.

Andrea, mother of Joya, age 3 months
Virginia

Everyone should pack a preemie outfit for pictures or for going home. (My son did not fit in any clothes, and he was 7 lbs. 4 oz.) All babies look swallowed up in their outfits in their hospital pictures. Also, take your own cute receiving blankets. I took my own polka-dotted ones, and my son's hospital pictures are cute.

Marie, mother of Cayden Marcus Dalme, age 4 months
Texas

Things to bring to the hospital: a pillow, so you can nurse your new baby in comfort; Tucks pads, so your bottom will be comfy; lots of extra underwear, because there's more bleeding than you would think; overnight sanitary napkins, because the hospital ones are not big enough. Be sure to write your name on all your personal items as well as "patient's own" so you don't get charged by the hospital for the things you brought from home.

Bekki, stay-at-home mother of Alec, age 16 months, and Baby #2 on the way
California

Don't stress out too much about what to bring with you to the hospital. Pack any basic items you might require and don't worry after that. Some items to pack might include a nursing bra, warm slippers and socks, a comfortable nightgown, and all standard toiletries such as a toothbrush, deodorant, a hair brush, etc. If you happen to need anything else while you're in the hospital (I forgot my toothbrush!), there's always someone ready and willing to go get it for you. Two things I was really glad I brought with me were my cell phone and lip balm — and they were both in my pocketbook.

Suzanne, teacher and mother of Sean, age 19, and Jennifer, age 14
New Jersey

Birth

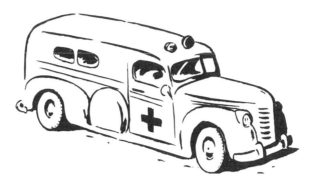

-Get Me to the Hospital-

No one told me to eat before I went to the hospital. I started going into labor when I woke up in the morning and went to the hospital. Fourteen hours later I could finally eat. Eat before you go.

Marie, mother of Cayden Marcus Dalme, age 4 months
Texas

Whether laboring or having a scheduled "C," try to at least put on some makeup or fix your hair before the baby comes. You will look better and enjoy the pictures much better in the time to come.

Leigh Donadieu, publisher of *Cuizine* magazine and mother of
Mitchell, age 4, and Ruth, age 2
New Jersey

Don't call family members when you're on your way to the hospital, especially if you're a first time parent. Many times you'll get to the hospital and, although you may be in labor, it's early labor, and you may be sent home. Be glad you're able to leave and be in a more comfortable place to labor. And it's less on your feelings of "adequacy" if you've never called anyone. Once you get to the hospital, have been checked cervically, and KNOW you're staying, then begin the phone calls.

JaLynn, mother of Kassie, age 14, and Kayla, age 7
Michigan

Are you in labor? You'll know when it starts! Trying to figure out when labor actually started was the hardest thing about being a first-time mom. I had no idea how I was supposed to know if this was the "real" thing or only Braxton-Hicks contractions. Guess what? You'll know! It will hurt more, and the contractions will come at regular intervals for a longer period of time.

Michele Braun Whiteaker, freelance writer and mother
Colorado

If you are planning on a hospital birth, then wait until active labor or when you feel like you can no longer handle the contractions before you go to the hospital. In active labor contractions are 4 minutes apart lasting 60 seconds or more. The further along you are in labor when you get to the hospital, the fewer unnecessary interventions; and the birth will be faster and the outcome better.

Candice, doula and mother of Skyler, age 5½, Sylvia, age 3, and Sage, age 1
California

Whether this is your first or fifth child, you will know that it is time for your baby to arrive. Do not be pushed out of the hospital and told to go home to wait it out. Walk around a bit, go to a local coffee shop, or rest in your car. My husband (this was his first child) and I went home, though my contractions were five minutes apart, and four hours later I gave birth in my bed with the paramedics, not in the birthing room as we had planned. There were no pictures or video, and my older daughter, who had gone to Lamaze with us and had been so excited about being present for the birth, was terrified. And my parents didn't make it on time. The worst part was that my husband called to tell my parents we had had the baby and were on the way to the hospital, but he did not specify which one. They assumed it would be the one we had planned to give birth in, but we were taken to the closest ER. When my parents showed up at my regular hospital, they were told that I had insisted on leaving. What a bunch of bologna! I was sick with a bad cold and having very painful contractions every five minutes, plus second babies typically come faster. Why would I want to leave?! My regular OB/GYN was very upset when he found out and asked why I had listened to the doctors and hadn't stayed around. Well, I told him I thought I could trust the MD's to tell me the right thing to do. I don't plan on having any more children. I am still suffering 2½ years later from major depression.

Diane, mother of Megan, age 11, and Molly, age 2½
California

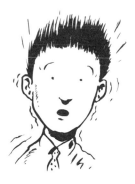

The Father-To-Be

Whether this is your first, second, or third baby, arrange to have not just your husband but a trusted girlfriend with you when you are in labor. While the actual birth you many want to share only with your husband, the sometimes LONG hours during the dialation part can be tough on a husband who often feels helpless to ease your pain. A trusted girlfriend (especially one who's already had a baby) can give your husband a break to get a bite to eat, brush his teeth, or take a rest without feeling guilty that he's abandoned you. My good friend and I played canasta while my husband walked to the deli across the street, had lunch, and when he can back he was refreshed and ready to help me through the pushing part. I wish I had done this with my first son, because when the pushing part came, my husband was so tired and hungry that he had a hard time mustering the enthusiasm I needed. With my second son, with the nice break he got thanks to my good friend Sabrina, he was more raring to go than I was!

Kellie, educator and mother of John, age 6, and Ian, age 3
Nevada

Assign everyone in your birth room a specific job. Grandmothers are great to "document" the birth by keeping a detailed record of what happened and when, and what people said and did – even writing a "Dear Baby" birth story to their grandchild when all is done. It will be a keeper for a lifetime, especially when the memories start to fade.

Jesse, childbirth educator, birth doula, and mother of Dashiell, age 1
Oregon

When in labor, try gazing into your partner's eyes as you breathe. Allow the love of your life to help you with delivery. Let him take an active role. I can hear you now: "He can't help me, I'm the one in labor." Well, actually he can. When your partner begins this process by being involved, the bonding of a new family goes much smoother. The need to "Get Dad Involved" after the baby is born isn't an issue. Dad has been there and active from the start. Here are a few ways you can accomplish this involvement.

Dad: You can tell whether Mom is tense or not during delivery by looking at her jaw, mouth, and the space between her eyebrows. When a woman is tense around her jaw and mouth area, then her pelvis is also tight. There is a connection! Midwives have used this tip for centuries! If Mom begins to wrinkle her brow, gently and with no words stroke her brow lightly as a signal to her to relax.

Mom: As you breathe, open your eyes and gaze into your partner's eyes. Allow him to absorb some of the waves of contractions.

Dad: Look into Mom's eyes and begin to use your imagination. Absorb some of the pain from her and then imagine it leaves your body and goes into the ground. You don't need it in your body either!

Mom: As you breathe use your imagination and make the connection to your cervix opening by giving yourself an image...maybe an infant's head coming out of a lotus blossom. With each breath you take imagine the cervix opening and your child's head coming through easily. Use whatever image you like to encourage cervical opening. You can also encourage opening to birth by allowing your body to sink into the waves of contractions versus pulling back from them. When you pull back from a contraction, you slow labor down. Labor will progress easier if you immerse yourself in the process instead of fighting it.

Look at it this way. Birth is simply the beginning of needing to immerse yourself in the parenting process. The sooner you learn to relax instead of fight the process, the easier family life is.

I've had the extraordinary privilege to give birth, naturally, to both of my sons. I've also been honored to attend three births as a doula. These tips worked for all five of the births.

Sharon Silver, founder and director of The Center for Conscious Parenting,
www.cfcp.info, and mother of two glorious young adults
Oregon

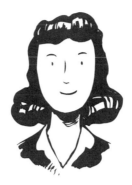

Helping Hands

A doula is a professionally trained childbirth assistant who provides emotional and physical support for a woman in labor. Statistics have shown that having a doula can help with having shorter labors, fewer cesareans, fewer complications, and needing less or no medication. There are also postpartum doulas who help with new-mom and newborn care. To learn more about doulas and to find one in your city, visit D.O.N.A. (Doulas of North America) at www.dona.org.

**Colleen, doula and childbirth educator and mother of
Emily, age 5, Alex, age 5, Celine, age 20 months, and Bryce, age 16 weeks
Arizona**

Make sure your opinion is heard while you're in the hospital. This is YOUR birth – your body, your baby, and your decisions. Be informed about what is being done to you, why, and ask for alternatives if you are uncomfortable. I've heard many moms express regret over not being forceful enough with hospital staff. However, I've never heard anyone say, "I'm sure glad I kept my opinions to myself and went along with something I didn't like." Remember – your body, your baby, your rights. You can even ask for a different doctor or nurse if you feel it's necessary.

**Kim, full-time mother of Tristen, age 3, and Josie, age 4 months
California**

Get a doula! First, it helps to have someone there to advocate for you and to also help your partner to help you in the best ways. Usually dads get frustrated and run out of ideas of ways to help mom during labor, and a doula is a great way to bridge that gap. Also, it's nice for the mom to have another woman there who can sympathize with what she's going through and reassure her that everything is fine, and she's doing great!

Shaana, doula and CBE and mother of
Nicholaus, age 20 months, and expecting Baby #2 in March 2005
California

Look into getting a doula. I couldn't have given birth without my husband there, but I also couldn't have done it without a doula. She was my liaison with the hospital attendants and was focused just on me. Check the DONA Web site for a doula near you.

Monica, stay-at-home mother of
Gus, age 9, Nathan, age 7, Emma, age 5, Carl, age 3, and Martin, age 1
Indiana

Having a doula present for your birth is the best way for you to know you'll have the necessary help in labor (physical, intellectual, and emotional), in addition to the support of your partner. Four hands are better than two, and a doula's knowledge and experience help make you more likely to cope with the pain, avoid unnecessary interventions and medications, and have a healthy and happy birth experience.

Jeanette, mother of Sophie, age 3½, and Miriam, age 10 months
Massachusetts

Hire a doula! My husband says "even if you're an obstetrician, hire a doula…because it's not about you." Our doula did whatever helped ALL of us…mother, baby, and father. When the entire medical staff was sure my induced labor would turn into a C-section, my doula kept that information from me and helped me to deliver a healthy 8-pound 14-ounce baby with no epidural, just as I'd hoped. Don't ever go through labor alone, even as a couple. Be sure to have a doula with you, too!

Laureen, teacher and mother of Jacob, age 5 months
Texas

The best thing I did with me second child was to hire a doula to help me with labor and delivery. My first labor was 33 hours long, and the nurses at the hospital were of no help and made no suggestions for speeding things up or making me more comfortable. With my second baby I decided the way to go was with the help of a doula. As well meaning as our husbands may be, it is much easier to listen to and follow the suggestions of a third party. My doula helped ease my back labor, got me what I needed in the hospital, and never interfered with my decisions. At a time when it's often hard to speak for yourself, a doula is a true advocate and comfort.

**Susan, women's medical supply company owner and mother of
Alex, age 6, and Hannah, age 18 months
California**

It's easy to feel bullied when you're half naked, exhausted, teary, and/or in pain. Try to have somebody with you (partner, sister, parent, friend) whom you trust to be your advocate and who won't be afraid to stand up to the members of the medical team. Medical personnel aren't necessarily great communicators; and you have a right to not only good care, but to understand the care you're receiving, to have your questions answered, and to have your wishes respected. Having somebody calm, assertive – even just mobile – to concentrate on your needs and act as your go-between can make a huge difference in your birth experience.

**Kristine, writer, editor, researcher, and mother of
Eleanor, age 22, and Emily, age 19
Illinois**

Use a doula for labor and postpartum support. The doula becomes a "tour guide" through labor, delivery, and birth by staying with you throughout your journey. She speaks the language and can help you reach your destination (delivery). A postpartum doula can help answer questions and support you and your family as you make the transition home. She can help with breastfeeding and can help take care of the home so mom can concentrate on taking care of herself and her baby. All new moms need help…don't be afraid to ask for it!

**Darla, labor doula, postpartum doula, childbirth educator, and mother of
Ashley, age 10, and Matthew, age 5
California**

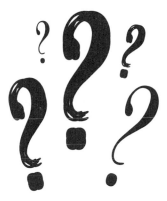

— Decisions to Make —

Research circumcision BEFORE your baby boy is born. The AAP no longer recommends it, and there are significant risks associated with it; so don't feel pressured into doing it if you don't feel like it's right for your baby!

**Kristin, mother of Conor, age 5 and born in a hospital, and
Bella, age 7 months and born at home in the water
Washington**

Do your research! Episiotomies are the leading cause of vaginal tears. In the absence of episiotomy, tears beyond a first degree, or rarely, a second degree, hardly ever occur. Ask your care provider to apply counterpressure when your baby is crowning and to keep the scissors away! An episiotomy is easier for the doctor to stitch but harder for you for healing. If you accept an episiotomy, you are trading a possible injury for a certain one. For what it's worth, I've had four children (all at home) — no episiotomies and no tears. Many doctors will tell you that they will decide if they are doing an episiotomy when the moment arises, but you can just outright refuse and state that you would rather tear.

**Elyssia, professional mother of
Samantha, age 8, Sophia, age 3, and Thomas and Iris, age 1**

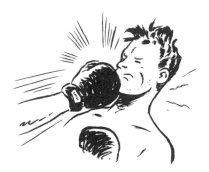

— Pain Management —

LOVED the epidural…that, along with music (Barenaked Ladies rocked William into this world!), made for a really fun birth experience.

Alicia, mother to William, age 1
New Jersey

I asked for a radio (now it would be a CD player) and tuned into my favorite music while in labor. It didn't take the labor pain away, but it did make it more bearable. Of course, if you're in labor in a cab or elevator, this may not work.

Barbara, professional "Mom Mom" and mother of Bill, age 34 and finally out of diapers, and Michael, age 32 and finally finished breast feeding
New Jersey

Spiral inward until you can go no further. Once you get there, get out of your own way and permit your body and breath to lead. Leave your judgement at home. It also helps to remember that the pain has a beginning and an end. Each contraction is a little mountain with the pain being worst at the precipice. Once you reach the peak of each contraction, the walk down the other side is like coming home.

Gail Silver, owner of Yoga Child and mother of Ben, age 5, and Anabel, age 3
Pennsylvania

I used an exercise ball during labour. It is a very large ball that you can sit on and rotate your pelvis. This is very helpful in assisting the baby's head through the pelvis. It is also great to rock backward and forward with the ball on all fours during contractions.

Sian, clinical nurse specialist and mother of Thomas, age 16,
Chelsea, age 12, Courtney, age 11, Caprice, age 6, and Chanelle, age 1
Cheshire, United Kingdom

God has a way of making a woman forget the true pain of childbirth. Thinking back on the births of my two children, all I remember is the beauty of the experience, not the pain. My best advice to a first time mom would be to not listen to others talk about the pain involved in childbirth. It is different for everyone, and I can assure you that any amount of pain is worth having once your beautiful baby is in your arms.

Melinda, mother of Sara, age 4, and Austin, age 2
Florida

What I know for sure about birth…I know that whatever kind of birth you are hoping for is possible. Your body was made to give birth and handle pain. Positive thinking and writing down your ideal birth experience is key to making it happen. It truly is mind over matter. It helps to have a loving support team, too. I know that seeing your baby for the first time is life changing, and it makes you forget about the pain.

Lea, courtesy of The Center for Conscious Parenting, www.cfcp.info,
mother of two little gems ages 3 and 2½ months
Oregon

For pain relief from contractions, try hot water. If your water hasn't broken and you are near a tub, or even a shower, hot water can be similar to morphine. I spent a couple of hours of my first labor in the bath, refilling it every so often with hot water. While I imagine there could be some small risks if you have high blood pressure or other health risks, most doctors and midwives will agree that the power of water to take the edge off of muscle contractions and the vicious pull of gravity is fantastic.

Ashley, mother of Flannery, age 9, and Gus, age 5
Tennessee

Childbirth is one of Nature's wonders, and each birth is unique: It is the beginning of life of a human being. Essential oils and flower essences such as Bach Flower Essences have been very useful both during labor and after birth to help both mother and child to adjust to each other and for the mother to get over the physical exhaustion of labor.

* Total panic and terrified of labor: Rock Rose, Rescue Remedy
* Fear of a known thing: Mimulus
* Fear of loosing control, not coping: Cherry Plum, Rescue Remedy
* Fear that something terrible is going to happen: Aspen
* Fear for the child: Red Chestnut
* Impatient for the labor to progress: Impatiens
* Exhaustion: Olive
* Lack of confidence: Larch

Four drops of Rescue Remedy in a glass of water sipped continuously throughout labor is very beneficial. Rescue Remedy contains Impatiens, Star of Bethlehem, Cherry Plum, Rock Rose, and Clematis.

**Bettina Rasmussen, co-owner of PlatyPaws Soft Soles Baby Shoes
and mother of Dylan, age 3
California**

Birth is the third of four stages of a woman's sexual maturity. During labor, walk, thrust your hips, dance, have an orgasm! Don't let anyone rush you! This all helps the process.

**Laura, mother of Nolan, age 14, and Neva, age 16 months
California**

Go through childbirth without drugs. It's good for babies and good to tell them when they are teenagers.

**Edna, high school teacher and mother of Sarah, age 23, and Allan, age 19
Texas**

During childbirth, instead of focusing on how bad it was, it was so helpful for me to be thankful that it wasn't worse. Somehow, that seemed to make it bearable, and I had three totally natural labors and deliveries. I have seen it work for some of my clients, too.

**MaryBeth, doula and mother of
Mikaela (stillborn), Jennifer, age 7, and Mason, age 3
Pennsylvania**

Stay out of bed! Women who labor upright and remain mobile have faster labors and experience less pain than those who restrict themselves to the bed.

Carol, birth attendant and mother of Robbie, age 5, and Windsor, age 2
Massachusetts

Leave the cape at home. Don't be a hero during your delivery. Surround yourself with people you trust and who respect your wishes, and then respect theirs. If you have watched too many baby stories on TV and have become rigid in your "delivery fantasy," let someone you trust tell you it's time to listen and consider option two. You have already achieved super hero status to someone very special...don't you just want to meet him/her?

Wendy, counselor and mother of
Katie, age 14 months, and second on the way
New Jersey

I have four children. With my first baby, I was totally naive and young and didn't know to ask for drugs. (This was 1968, so I don't even know if epidurals were available then.) With the second I was too dilated to get any pain relief medication. During my third pregnancy, my OB told me he was going to order an epidural, and I accepted his decision, no questions asked. During my first appointment with the fourth pregnancy, I told HIM I wanted an epidural. (Why should I deal with the pain if I didn't have to?) How I delivered each baby had no effect on how I bonded or loved them. The ability to endure pain has absolutely nothing to do with your worth as a mother.

Joanne, editor and mother of four and grandmother of four
New Jersey

I am extremely modest and was mortified at the thought of having so many people staring at my crotch during labor and delivery. I was even more worried about the possibility of having a bowel movement while pushing. I was actually much more worried about these things during my pregnancy than I was about labor and pain! When the time came, my little phobias became godsends. Obsessing over my fears actually helped take my mind off the real pain during labor! And, thankfully, I did not poop.

Anonymous (for obvious reasons), mother of one cute, very immodest 2-year-old
Wyoming

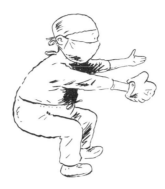

–Labor & Vaginal Birth–

My military husband half-jokingly offered this insight from his parachute jumping training. "Free you mind and your ass will follow."

Joe's wife, mother of Christopher and Katherine
Wisconsin

Here's a pushing tip that only your girlfriends will tell you about. This will probably sound crude. This tip was the best advice anyone ever gave me when it came time to get that (very large) baby out, and I am grateful to this day that she shared it with me. As you are laying there in that most undignified position and the doctor tells you to push, concentrate on shooting your butt across the room. Yes, that's right – you're using the same muscles that you use for a bowel movement (which will likely happen during labor, too, in case no one has let you know that), and you pretty much have to pretend you are taking the biggest poop of your life. Sorry ladies, but it's the truth, and it works.

Jennifer, part-time director of community relations and mother of
Grace, age 3½, and Anna, age 10 months
Iowa

Don't be afraid to own your birth experience. When we surrender to the awesome power of birth, it becomes more manageable and happens a lot faster.

Kimberly, birth doula and mother of Jacob, age 4, and Keenan, age 2
Illinois

Be sure to talk to your doctor prior to labor about which muscles you should use for "pushing" during natural childbirth. A friend explained it to me and, being pregnant for the first time, it was something that I had never given a second thought. Prior to that conversation I truly believed that you should push with your "stomach muscles." I'd seen it on TV a million times...

Kim, mother of Blake, age 3
California

You've read all the books, attended childbirth classes, subscribed to the magazines, and talked to your friends and family about their experiences. The thing is, no one tells you what you really need to know. For instance, everyone's experience is different! Here's a few things to remember.

1. It's messy, messy, messy! Do you envision the birth of your child just like it happens on TV? Wearing full makeup, you'll do a lot of huffing and puffing, maybe say something nasty to your husband, and out pops your baby. Guess again. I'll spare you by not going into too much detail, but imagine fluids exploding from every orifice of your body at the same time!

2. Don't wear your own nightgown. How many articles advise you to wear your own nightshirt? Some childbirth instructors stress this as one of the most important aspects of the birthing experience: "You shouldn't feel like property of the hospital," they say. See #1 above! Hopefully the nurse on duty will persuade you to wear a hospital gown. Although not glamorous, at least it's soft and practical.

3. Consider having more than one support person. Some people won't feel comfortable with this option, but it worked great for me. My husband, mother, and sister were all there to help me through labor. It allowed my husband to take breaks, and I needed all three when it came time to push. I had my husband holding one leg, my sister clamped onto the other, and my mom rooting me on over the doctor's shoulder.

Michele Braun Whiteaker, freelance writer and mother
Colorado

"Let your uterus do all the work" is key...don't fight labor. Work on keeping your body and mind relaxed so your uterus can do the whole thing for you.

Jeanette, mother of Sophie, age 3½, and Miriam, age 10 months
Massachusetts

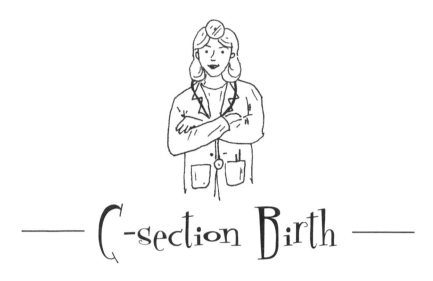

C-section Birth

As a mom of two, a birth doula, and a childbirth educator, I didn't think I would ever end up having a C-section. However, my third delivery ended up being a cesarean! It was still a great birth. I made sure I had music of my choice playing in the delivery room; and when I got my first glimpse of my son, I had my husband unwrap him and lay him on my chest so I could touch and feel him right away. It wasn't what I had expected, but I had planned for the unexpected and was ready with the choices that were important to me.

Erica, RN, doula, childbirth educator, and mother of
Josh, age 6, Zach, age 4, and Ben, age 16 months
Minnesota

Most hospitals put the baby in the nursery for observation immediately following a C-section. However, if your baby's apgar score is good at birth, you can request to have your baby straight away (providing you are awake) and put him/her to the breast as soon as possible. I have had all four children via C-section, all nursed within minutes of birth, and it sure gets breastfeeding off to a wonderful start. Good communication between you and your nurses and doctors is vital. Let them know what's important to you.

Maureen
Vancouver, Canada

Best baby invention for a C-section delivery? Two words…Boppy Pillow! It helped me so much when I couldn't lift my son right away, and it didn't hurt my incision site either. I used it when he got to be a few months old to help him sit up, too! My son used it for a long time. He even digs it out now and then and lays on it as a pillow when he's watching a movie or taking a nap. I highly suggest that all new moms get or register for a Bobby Pillow!

Nicole, special events coordinator for March of Dimes and mother of Ashton, age 16 months
Wisconsin

Be prepared for your nurse to completely bathe and clean you several times in the first 24 to 48 hours. It is embarrassing, but being prepared helps.

Lavette, mother of Evy, age 1
South Carolina

My mother, who had recently recovered from a hysterectomy, gave me this incredibly helpful advice. She said no matter how much you feel like walking doubled over, cradling your belly in your arms, don't. Stand up straight, stretching your abdomen up tall and cultivate the posture your mother always wanted you to have. You will heal faster, have less pain, move with greater ease, and even though it might feel like your guts are going to fall out, they won't! It was true for me.

Pam, consultant and mother of Zach, age 18
Washington

Honestly, it wasn't that bad. The surgery itself was far easier than the contractions that preceded it. Afterward, it is important to listen to the nurses. Make sure you get up when they tell you and walk around, even though you will be scared to death to do so. Recovery was relatively easy after the first day (much easier than I had imagined, actually). I have friends who WANTED elective C-sections and couldn't get them. So remember, if you have one, someone out there is jealous.

Connie, publisher and mother of Holden, age 3
New Jersey

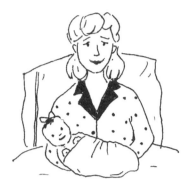

Afterward

Don't worry and get upset with yourself if you don't bond right away with your baby or experience overwhelmingly sentimental maternal feelings. Many women don't bond in those first few days or weeks because they are going through such a huge transition, and everyone reacts to it differently and bonds at their own pace. Remember, love comes from giving. As time passes and you give more and more to your baby, that love, bond, and closeness will grow and flourish.

**Sarah Zeldman, Life Balance coach – Balanced Woman Coaching,
www.Balanced-woman-coaching.com,
and mother of Yosef, age 3½, and Shanya, age 1
New York**

After years of working with pregnancy-related publications, reading all the materials that I could find regarding childbirth during my first pregnancy, and having spent hours listening closely to friends and family as they shared their birthing experiences, I was so blindly confident that I was "prepared" for childbirth that I was crushed when things didn't work out as I had planned. Although I firmly believe childbirth "preparation" is extremely important, I realized that a baby cannot read the "birth plan" and that an open mind and prayer are sometimes the only ways to handle what life throws at you!

**Debora Robertson, group publication manager – *Expectant Mother's Guide* series
and mother of Adam, age 3½, and Anna, age 10 months
Pennsylvania**

When the midwife or doctor gives you your baby that you have been waiting nine months to see, demand that you hold him/her so that you can bond. I cannot think of any newborn procedure that can't wait until you have looked into you newborn's eyes and looked him/her over from head to toe. That is where your baby feels safest, on your chest, not being weighed or poked or frightened away from you, the only thing he/she recognizes in this new scary world.

Layla, certified birth doula and mother of Brandon, age 16, Alasyn, age 11, Colton, age 10, Andy, age 9, Shadd, age 8, Tyler, age 6, and Ethan, age 3
Oregon

Bonding is so important. I think one of the best things to do when you are feeding or changing or just spending time with your new baby is to try to focus all you attention on your baby. Talk to baby, explain what you are doing, and sing, even if you don't think you have a good voice. I guarantee your baby thinks it's the best voice he/she has ever heard. Get lost in your baby's eyes several times a day. Get a routine so things are not so stressful. If you are stressed, your baby will also be stressed, and then you will not have a happy baby. Enjoy your baby the best that you can.

Dawn, RN, and mother of Sophia, age 3, and Analiese, age 1
New Jersey

At least twenty percent of new moms experience postpartum depression. It is a very serious illness but is totally treatable. My tip is it is vitally important to make sure you are well educated about risk factors, symptoms, and where to go for treatment should PPD effect you. For more information, visit www.ppdsupport.org, and www.postpartum.net.

Helena Bradford, Chm., The Ruth Craven Foundation for Postpartum Depression Awareness
South Carolina

If your labor and delivery didn't go exactly as you had hoped, get all the details from someone else who was there. As a birth coach, I've found that many women think they're remembering exactly what happened, but they weren't aware of everything. Once they get additional information, they can understand why certain interventions were taken. Then, they feel less disappointed and more positive about their birth experience.

Sheryl Gurrentz, author of *The Guilt-Free Guide to Your New Life as a Mom* and *If Your Child is Bipolar* and mother of Jordan, age 13, and Joey, age 10
Colorado

Don't expect to immediately fall in love with your baby on Day 1. It's like any relationship: sometimes it takes a few weeks or months to fall in love.

Kate, writer and mother of Jude, age 3, and Belle, age 6 months

My son came down with jaundice while we where still in the hospital. The remedy the nurses had was for me not to breastfeed him but to let them keep him in the nursery and bottle feed him at very specific intervals. This felt funny to me, but I was just a new mom, and they were professionals, so I didn't question it – I just accepted it. After going home, talking with mothers, and reading more on jaundice, I learned that breastfeeding is much better for a baby with jaundice. My tip is don't be afraid to question things that just don't feel right. I really wish I had.

**Kimberly, BA child development and mother of Alexander, age 1
California**

During the birth of my first son Lucas, I had an episiotomy as he was so big! I felt let down and depressed during the recovery after birth as midwives and doctors prepare for the nine months pregnancy and labour, but no advice is given about after the birth, recovery, and how you might feel. It was hard for me, and my tip for new mothers would be to make time for yourself as soon as possible, pamper yourself, even if it's a long quiet soak in the bath; and remember it will get better, and there is support out there! Don't shut yourself away. Get out and show that baby off!!

**Wendy, qualified nanny and mother of Lucas, age 2
Basingstoke, United Kingdom**

Straight after giving birth and for about two weeks after, I said I would never, ever do it again; and it really scared me because, at the time, I meant it and hadn't been expecting to feel like that. My poor newborn, who was beautiful, was going to be an only child, because I couldn't bear to go through that same experience again! Two weeks later I was saying, "When I have the next one…" I went on to warn all of my friends that this would probably happen to them (which it did) so that they didn't worry about those feelings like I did! I just wish someone had warned me!

Lisa, nanny and mother of Jack, age 23 months

That Lamaze breathing, HONEY…you don't need this for labor –
you'll need this for when you're trying to deal with your
toddler…hoo hoo hoo, hee hee hee.

**Tina, bookkeeper and mother of
Fisher, age 5, Eli, age 2, and Sullivan, age 9 months
Texas**

If you are a mother with type O blood and your baby's father has a
different blood type, educate yourself about ABO incompatibility jaundice
of the newborn, also called "abnormal jaundice." This condition is easily
abated with light therapy, but can be detected earlier by certain blood
tests immediately after the birth if your baby might be at risk.

**Diana, professional clarinetist and mother of
Anna, age 2, and newborn Simon
New York**

Don't plan for anything and throw away those "Birth Plans." I
wanted a natural water birth and ended up with a 62 hour labor (and
back labor), augmented with Pitocin for 24 hours and epidural for
the last 12, followed by a cesarean section because my baby was OP
and deflexed and would not turn around. Water completely stopped
my uterus from contracting, and it seemed like nothing could get
that boy out. But now we've got him, and he is wonderful.

**Jennifer, computer technology instructor and mother of
Nicholas, age 2½ weeks
Oregon**

After the baby is born, the only thing that will be consistent in your
life will be inconsistency. As soon as you realize and accept that,
you will be a much happier parent.

**Jacque, CLE and mother of Kyleigh, age 8, and Karissa, age 4½
California**

Lots of new moms have times when they feel frustrated, out of
control, and resentful. If you feel this way, it doesn't mean that you
aren't a good mom. It just means that you're a normal new mom!

**Sheryl Gurrentz, author of *The Guilt-Free Guide to Your New Life as a Mom* and
If Your Child is Bipolar and mother of Jordan, age 13, and Joey, age 10
Colorado**

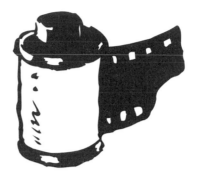

First Memories

Keep a journal from Day One. Even if you're not a writer, just scribble down a few thoughts every day. The world will seem so upside down, you can't remember your name. You'll want to remember some of the cute little things that happen. I think I treasure my journal more than the baby book or photo albums. It holds memories that would be quickly forgotten had I not recorded them in a journal.

Michele Braun Whiteaker, freelance writer and mother
Colorado

If possible, video as much as possible of your labor and birth as you can. If you never ever watch it or only watch it once, you will always have the option to see it or save it if you want to. You could even destroy it if it is too much to keep. But if you don't make some sort of recording of the event, even the "gross" stuff, you can never get a do over. Granted, you might have more babies down the road, but THAT child's birth is a onetime deal. Don't miss it. You'll want to see it more than you think!

Stacy Walker, wellness encourager, www.Manna4Me.com, and mother of
Shayne, age 8, Harris Anne, age 6, David, age 4, and Hudson, age 1
Alabama

At age 33, I found myself expecting quadruplets. Already a mother of one daughter, who was almost 13, I was a little unprepared for experiences I was going to endure. Thankfully, we had many friends and family ready and willing to take pictures of me during my pregnancy and after as well. Have many cameras on hand. Take pictures; do not worry about how you look in the moment. When you show the pictures to those children you were carrying at the time, their excitement becomes very contagious. We delivered the quads 10 weeks early, and I developed toxemia after the delivery. I am forever grateful to the wonderful nursing staff at the UIHC NICU for their quick thoughts. They took pictures of all four of our babies and gave them to my husband so he could share them with me since I had to stay in bed. The kids are now 5 going on 6, and I am still very happy with the quick thinking of all involved for remembering to get pictures of the kids for me.

Debbie, mother of Krystle, age 18, Kassidy, age 5, Allen, age 5, Aaran, age 5, and Andrew, age 5
Iowa

Take a special journal to the hospital and, while there, take the time to write down a few of your feelings about the birth and your thoughts about the new baby now in your family. Though a new mom does not have a lot of spare time, the journal is a way to preserve some thoughts, memories, and even classic lines the children come up with as they get older. When they are grown, you can have a little bit more information for them than that "first tooth" or "first step." If you have more than one child, they will each have their own storybook of treasured thoughts and feelings.

Nancy, RN, childbirth educator, doula, and mother of four boys ages 15 to 26
Maryland

Take a picture of your child on his/her monthly "birthday," starting the day of his/her birth, and then once a month on his/her "birthday" throughout the first year. It is truly wonderful to look back over the first year and see how much your child has grown and changed. Your heart warms even more, and you see how much you are nurturing this little person you helped create and bring into this world.

Laila, work-at-home business consultant and mother of Maria, age 2, and Matthew, age 4 months
British Columbia, Canada

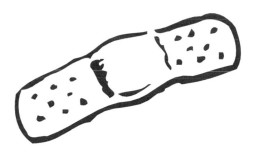

Postpartum Care

How to help a sore perineum: Wet paper towels and fold them into the size of a panty liner. Freeze. Take out one at a time and wrap it in a dry paper towel. Place it in your underwear like a pad. You have the comfort of an ice pack without the bulk of one. They don't cost a lot. When it gets warm, you can throw it away. Save your ice packs for the beach.

**Micheline, doula, childbirth educator, lactation consultant,
day care provider, and mother of 3
British Columbia, Canada**

Try a JAASON product called Witch-Vera. After a vaginal birth, use this on your pad. It helps with everything from hemorrhoids to episiotomies. It feels great, and it helps you heal twice as fast!

**Susan, doula and mother of Bella, age 5, and Sophia, age 3
New York**

Ask the maternity ward if they will provide the special maxi pads with a built-in cold pack. I had a very difficult delivery, requiring an episiotomy, and the "cold" maxi pads were incredibly soothing to my sore and swollen perineum. If your hospital does not stock them, buy them online beforehand!

**Kate, advertising account supervisor and mother of Jackson, age 4 months
Pennsylvania**

Stuff cold cabbage leaves in your bra after your milk comes in (whether you breastfeed or not) to help relieve engorgement. No one seems to know why it works, but it helped me so much, considering I found engorgement more painful than the actual birth of either of my kids.

**Tracy, director of Christian education and mother of
Hannah, age 2, and Christian, age 4 months
Pennsylvania**

If you have stitches after birth, take some salt and bathe stitches with a salt water solution every time you go to the toilet. This helps keep stitches infection free.

**Tamalyn Roberts, Web site owner, www.names2be.com, and mother of
Natalie, age 9, Matthew, age 7, and Paul, age 5
Anglesey, United Kingdom**

After birthing, cold packs will be a big comfort to your vaginal area. Here's an easy way to make some for home: In a baking pan, lay maxi pads side by side. Pour a bottle of witch hazel over them and put the pan in the freezer. When you want a cold pack, you'll be ready!

**Sandy, physical therapist and mother of Marika, age 4, and Haley, age 1
California**

One thing that I don't believe I could have lived without during those first few weeks after birth was the herbal afterbirth sitz bath. You can buy it at any health food store. (It will have directions on how to prepare the bath.) It really helps to heal any vaginal tears and is just plain heavenly. Give the baby to your partner for 20 minutes while you enjoy this time to take care of yourself.

**Susan, mother of Athena, age 16 months
Colorado**

You still go through contractions after the birth! Sometimes, quite painful ones! I didn't know that you still get the contractions after the baby is born. Keep lots of Tylenol on hand and have lots of patience!

**Trisha, stay-at-home mother of Emily Faith, age 8 months
Manitoba, Canada**

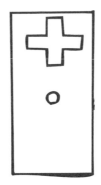

—Days in the Hospital—

It was very important to me to include my first born in the birth of our second as much as possible. On my hospital door, I scrapbooked a page of pictures of my 4-year-old welcoming our new baby. The hospital staff would always comment, and this would make our 4-year-old feel real special.

Stephanie, counselor LPC and mother of Jack, age 4, and Will, age 1½
Oklahoma

If you are naming your child after a meaningful relative or friend, consider including that information on the birth announcement. For example: Benjamin Leo is named in loving memory of his great-grandfather, Leo. This way, you can share your joyful news while paying tribute to a special person in your life whom you'll want your child to know about one day.

Debbie Glasser, Ph. D., licensed clinical psychologist, founder of NewsForParents.org, and mother of Emily, age 12, Benjamin, age 8, and Sam, age 2
Florida

The hospital took an imprint of my baby's foot after he was born. We scanned it into the computer and printed off thank-you cards that had his foot on the front of the card and his name underneath.

Amy Tardio, therapist, counselor, and mother of John, age 1
Illinois

After living on ice chips and slushies for almost 36 hours and feeling like I'd run a marathon, all I wanted was food. Hospital food didn't cut it either! My menus somehow got switched with the mommy next door and her tastes were the polar opposite of mine. In my foggy state, it took me two meals to figure this out, and by then I was almost checked out of the hospital. My sister-in-law was a lifesaver when she thought to bring me a steaming hot chicken pot pie, plate of mashed potatoes, and berry cobbler from my favorite restaurant. My hero!

Michele Braun Whiteaker, freelance writer and mother
Colorado

In addition to pillaging both in-hospital bassinets for all the baby bookable "It's a Boy"/"It's a Girl"/"I'm a Twin!" stickers, signs, and test results, when leaving the hospital be sure to ask for any "freebies" or extra supplies they are willing to pass along. Formula companies and diaper manufacturers usually have "gifts" for the new baby(ies) waiting at the hospital for you. Don't be shy; ask for what's available.

Cheryl Lage, Web host of www.twinsights.com, a site for new and expecting twin
moms, and full-time mother of fraternal twins, Darren and Sarah Jane, age 3
Virginia

Do not be afraid to say no to visitors, including your family. In the first few days after the baby is born, you will need your rest as well as quality time to spend bonding with your baby. You will also need to adjust to the change in your lifestyle. Visitors will sometimes cause undue stress as well as create resentment as you may feel that you need to entertain them or let them hold the baby. Do not leave it up to your husband to say something, because often times he won't!

Lucille, mother of Nicholas, age 2
New York

Bring a blank book, scrapbook, or just some loose pieces of paper to the hospital and have visitors and special hospital staff sign it. Believe it or not, you will forget so much of what happens the first few days, and it's nice to have a record of the people who were with you.

Stacy, graphic artist, owner of Inkspot Creations, and mother of Julia, age 18 months
New Jersey

─Breastfeeding Opinions─

Breastfeeding is not for everyone – and it's up to YOU to make the decision. Your baby benefits no matter what you choose: don't breastfeed (there are a gazillion choices of excellent formula out there), do a 50/50, or breastfeed exclusively. Why? Because you are holding that little miracle and singing or talking to him or her and nurturing him or her. And I say nurturing because the body, the heart, and the mind are involved for the both of you. You do what's best for the both of you because in the long run, at the 2:30 AM feeding, that's what counts.

Karina, teacher and mother of Ben, age 18, and Ilana, age 16
Maryland

Breast is best, but if it's not for you, don't be guilted into it by anyone. It doesn't matter how you feed your baby, just that you feed your baby.

Dawn, RN, and mother of Sophia, age 3, and Analiese, age 1
New Jersey

There is nothing in this entire world as beautiful as the pair of eyes that look into yours as you feed your baby. Nothing is as beautiful to them as when you hold them close to feed them and sing them a lullaby.

Milynda, social worker and mother of Leif, age 16, and Mackinley, age 13
Michigan

Many of our moms have sent in tips about breastfeeding and the importance of doing so. I breastfed my four children, and indeed, it was a wonderful experience. However, there are many circumstances when breastfeeding may not be possible: a must-work situation for a single parent or a financially strapped couple; a working mom/stay-at-home dad arrangement; severed mammary ducts caused by medically mandated breast reduction surgery; physical impairments – to name a few. A mom, especially a first-time mom, should not be made to feel guilty or less motherly because her baby is being fed formula from a bottle instead of milk from a breast. Your baby will still be held/cuddled, nurtured, nourished, and will thrive. Over the years I have had the pleasure of bottle feeding other people's babies, including three of my grandchildren (!), and you know what? Babies react the same way whether breastfed or bottle fed. They look at you, play with your fingers, reach for your face, make cooing/gurgly sounds, SMILE. Their little tummies are getting full – life is good!

Joanne, editor and mother of four and grandmother of four
New Jersey

When I was pregnant with my son Issac, one of the first questions anyone asked me was "Are you going to breastfeed?" I researched it and planned on breastfeeding – "the breast is the best." Well, things don't always work out as planned. When I had Issac, I was physically unable to breastfeed my son. Within 12 hours of being a new mom I already felt like a failure. I failed at my first job as a mom. My advice to any new mom who faces this is not to feel like a failure. Write a list of the PROS of formula feeding (i.e., Daddy could help with the feedings; Daddy can share in the late night feedings; no nursing bras or nursing pads to wear; NO LEAKING). Focus on the good, surround yourself with support, and realize that your baby will be just as happy and healthy without the breast milk. What's really important is the love you give to your new precious bundle.

Rachelle, legal assistant and mother of Issac, age 6 months
Oklahoma

After you deliver, be sure to breastfeed your little one – it's best for him/her and for you. Breastfed is bestfed. And definitely buy and apply lots of Lansinoh cream. You'll probably feel like your nipples are on fire after a day or two. It's a lifesaver!

Mary, small business owner and stay-at-home mother of
Jennie, age 5½, and Michael, age 2½
New Jersey

Many moms waver on the subject of nursing vs. formula, but let me tell you, for me nursing is an absolute joy. Your body is producing the most nutritious, perfect food for your baby. It's always the right temperature, and it's always the right amount. It's the perfect food when your baby is ill. It's portable, environmentally friendly, and has numerous health benefits over formula. Trust your body; it knows what to do – breastfeed! It's easier than you can even imagine and endlessly fulfilling.

**Kim, full-time mother of Tristen, age 3, and Josie, age 4 months
California**

I have always believed that the decision to breastfeed is a very personal one. I am the mother of three, and, for me, breastfeeding was something I always knew I'd do. Physically, you have to be prepared for those first few days. Yes, in some cases, you may have some pain and discomfort. But after dealing with nine months of throwing up, heartburn, weight gain, and praying that whatever is growing out of your tush disappears, are we not warriors? With my oldest I remember having minimal discomfort and he being a great feeder. My second child also took well to breastfeeding, but I discovered that the uterus contractions caused when the baby sucked were not pleasant. Of course, if you keep in mind that studies have shown that this helps the uterus to contract back to its normal size faster, this may help you to focus. By the time I had my third child, I thought I was a breastfeeding pro. Wrong. He latched on like a baby piglet at an eating marathon with the strength of an industrial vacuum. The contractions I experienced could only be compared to mini labors (no epidural). For me, this was the point when I looked down at my nipples that looked like big throbbing raspberries, felt contractions that made me want to cry, and encountered nausea (Did I mention the nausea?); and I thought, I'm doing this, why? But the why was right there in my arms; and as I looked down at him, I knew that the choice to breastfeed was not a choice but a commitment that we make to our children. That is the commitment to give our children the best start possible. I have been fortunate to be able to breastfeed each of my children. I have enjoyed the closeness and the bond that I feel breastfeeding gives, not to mention the health benefits to the child. When all is said and done, whether you breastfeed or go with formula, enjoy your children, do your best by them, and you will be rewarded no end.

**Lourdes, mother of Ricky, age 20, Suzzel, age 14, and Julian, age 23 months
California**

Best thing to do is breastfeed: totally convenient, always available, exactly the nutritional mix needed for a human baby. The World Health Organization recommends breastfeeding for two years at least. If you're scared that you won't be able to do it, call La Leche League and go to a meeting or get a home visit! Nature's convenience food!

Sarah, civil engineer and mother of a little boy, age 2½
New York

Breastfeed your baby. Read books. Talk to moms who have successfully breastfed their children. Contact La Leche League or your birthing center. Get help latching baby on correctly. If it hurts, you need to break suction and try again! Tell your husband how much money he will save now (no need for artificial baby milk) and in the future (healthier children!).

Pat McGough-Wujcik, drummer for The Mydols and mother of
Megan, age 19, Nick, age 12, Ryan, age 10, and Sophy, age 4
Michigan

If you formula fed a previous baby or think formula feeding is the way to go, start out breastfeeding anyway! It's so much easier to switch to the bottle at 8 weeks or so, if you still want to do that, than to relactate and breastfeed a couple months down the road! The colostrum the baby gets in the first hours of life is crucial to completing the immune system and flushing out meconium. The sucking action of the baby is great for shrinking the uterus back to size and helps mom lose a chunk of her "baby fat." Babies often want to be right on mom for at least the first couple of months, and no other care provider makes them happier! Breastfeeding is easier than bottle feeding because all the supplies are already on mom. At 6 weeks or so, see how you feel about feeding the baby, but know that the choice is easier now than prior to meeting your little one.

Kate, biologist and mother of Ursula, age 9, Sage, age 7, and Benno, age 3
Colorado

It is okay if you want to breastfeed, AND it is okay if you use formula. As long as your baby is happy and his/her needs are met, that is what is important. And don't feel guilty about stopping breastfeeding: everyone is different.

Lori, advertising project manager and mother of Lincoln, age 18 months

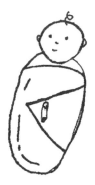

—Life in the NICU—

If your baby is born prematurely and you have to spend time in the NICU, be sure to keep hands-on contact with your baby, no matter how fragile he/she seems. A preemie needs to be touched and held just as much as any other baby.

Eleanor, journalism student and mother of Sophia, age 19 months
Illinois

Do not worry about how much milk you pump…even the smallest amount will help your baby.

Laura, party and gift consultant and mother of Claire, age 5

Be positive and focus on the little things. When our little one was in the NICU, we kept a journal of her progression; and if you read the journal today, you won't find a word about complication or medical concern, only the simple things in life that are an accomplishment for a NICU baby. Being constantly obsessed with the medical concerns will drag you down and burn you out quickly. Our child was so premature we got to focus on things like opening her eyes for the first time, a first feeding, even a first bowel movement. Anything that is an accomplishment for your little one is where you should focus.

Jennifer, LVN and mother of Sarah Louise
Colorado

I guess there are so many tips to give anyone who has had a premature birth. After our son was born at 24 weeks (1 pound and 3 ounces) in a different state that we were visiting, we learned a lot during his 11-month hospital stay. But I think the best tip we could give is to never underestimate the strength and will of a baby, no matter how small. Babies are stronger then you know. Also, be there: not just stand and be there, but be there for every second that they fight to live; each moment they struggle to breathe. Stay in touch, talk to and keep in constant contact with not only your baby, but with the doctors, nurses, and other families as well. Full family support was why our Robbie survived a fight that he was not supposed to win. He was at death's door so many times that death gave up on him. We made sure he knew we were there, we gave him reasons to live, and we made promises that we promised to keep. Along with support and love we said a lot of prayers. We had never prayed so much in our lives as we did in those 11 months! Love your baby no matter what and never give up, stop believing, or stop having faith. Never underestimate the strength or the will of a baby. He gave us strength to be strong. One so little had led our way. God bless.

Beth, mother of Kenneth, age 14, Kendra, age 13, and Robbie, age 2½
Missouri

Even though the NICU is a frightening place, it is very important to get comfortable and to make the most of the critical time your baby is there. Don't be shy about spending time bedside. I sat in a glider with a book or journal all day, every day. I did not bother the nurses, but I did befriend them and asked periodically if I could lower the side of the layette so I could lay my head next to my baby for a bit of a cuddle. If they need to intervene or perform other ministrations on your baby, stay out of the way or leave the room, if possible. Give them space to do their jobs and always remember that they are saving your baby's life and trying to send you home with a whole, healthy child. Don't fuss about shaved heads or blown veins. If the doctors and nurses are not worried about having to care for you as well as your child, they will be happy to have you there and will help you learn about what is happening. Be strong. Be grateful. Love your baby. And send pictures later so they can see the result of their efforts. They so often only see the sick children, and it helps them to see your child happy and well later on. Never forget the good people who took care of your child.

Mindy, nonprofit manager and mother of
Logan, age 6½, Dylan, age 4, and Daphne, age 2½
California

Tiny babies need you to believe. If you are their mom or dad, another relative, a friend from work, a passerby, a nurse or doula, a painter, an insurance salesman, or a grocery store checker even who hears their name – they need you to believe that inside their tiny little hearts is a passion for LIFE. Call out to them and bring it forth. You will never be the same.

**Courtney, nurturing labor doula to mother of Baby A,
who was born at 28 weeks gestation and responded to the call to LIFE
Texas**

Skin-to-skin or Kangaroo care is well documented to enhance and speed the growth of premature babies. This is essential to full-term infants as well. Breastfeeding provides some skin-to-skin contact. Sleeping on a naked daddy's chest, bathing together, or infant massages are all forms of this brain developing essential contact.

**Mary, PA, IBCLC, and mother of
Michael, age 27, Susan, age 27, and Elizabeth, age 22
Idaho**

Touch and hold your baby skin to skin as often as it is allowed. He/ She will feel it and recognize you. You will be greatly rewarded for it with increased attachment and possibly an earlier release.

**Mary, professor and mother of Sean, age 10 months
Illinois**

When you are the mom of a preemie, remember to get lots of sleep when you can. It will help you in the long run.

**Laura, party and gift consultant and mother of Claire, age 5
Colorado**

Listen to the doctors but pay attention to the nurses! And look at your baby, not the monitor! (They had to cover the monitor for me!) You'll learn to read your baby that way.

**Michelle, teacher and mother of
Tyler, age 17 months, born at 30 weeks and met by his adopted parents at 2 days old
California**

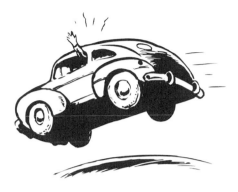

Going Home

If you're going to be in a SUV or another high vehicle when you leave the hospital after a C-section or a rough vaginal delivery, make sure the person picking you up brings a stool so it's easier for you to climb into the vehicle.

Sheryl Gurrentz, author of *The Guilt-Free Guide to Your New Life as a Mom* and *If Your Child is Bipolar* and mother of Jordan, age 13, and Joey, age 10
Colorado

My oldest son was born with hydrocephalus and had a mechanical draining device placed in his skull four days after birth. After nine days the doctor discharged him and told us to take him home. I looked at her and said, "What do I do with him?" thinking I had to treat him differently because of his surgery. Her response helped to shape our relationship that continues today. "Just love him," she said simply.

Kim, mother of Elias, age 4, Rhett, age 2½, and Sloan, age 8 months
Arkansas

Labor is the easy part. The next 20 years are the hard work. Relax and enjoy the ride.

Susie, RN, and mother of Christopher, age 21, and Molly, age 20

Baby's First Year

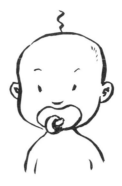

─── Baby's First Days ───

For the first 6 weeks of your baby's life, it is important to swaddle (wrap like a burrito) because babies have no control over their arms and legs. This will help to control their body parts and get good sleep. They feel as snug and safe as when they were in the womb.

**Valerie Ybarra, baby nurse, postpartum doula,owner www.babynurseonthego.com,
and mother of Alexis, age 15, and Arianna, age 8
Georgia**

Remember that your newborn is very knowledgeable about the things that matter in the beginning. Newborns know how to find your breast, how to latch on, how to time sucking, swallowing, and breathing. They know when they are hungry and when they have had their fill. They know your voice, smell, and how to call you and mobilize you to help them get what they need. When you are trying to manage being a new mom, it can be a relief to remember that your newborn is a knowledgeable and active person, too. You are a team, and you are both doing the best you can.

Karen, Ph.D., translator and mother of Ingrid, age 5

Listen to your heart, not your head. HOLD and CUDDLE your new baby as much as you can. Food "spoils," babies "thrive."

**Barb, retired and mother of Jonas, age 25
Washington**

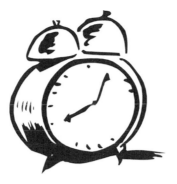

— Baby's Schedule —

It is so important to set a routine for your baby. Remember that you are the boss, not your baby. To establish the schedule, your baby will have to cry it out on more than one occasion. This will hurt you more than the baby. Be strong and stick to your routine and schedule.

Rachelle, mother of Kagan, age 2
Texas

We used a sleep schedule from a very early age for our son and noticed a huge difference between our son and other children his age. He was happy, alert, and pleasant to be around. Rarely did he fuss because he was always well rested. Sometimes it was a bit of a hassle to run my life around his napping, but it was all worthwhile because we had a baby that was fun to be with. We continue the nap schedule today (he's 17 months) and think that napping is the key to a happy child who is ready to learn and fun to be with.

Elisa, management consultant and mother of Quinn, age 17 months
Colorado

To avoid frustration — and keep your sanity — remember that, for awhile at least, you are on your baby's schedule. Frustration only sneaks in when you try to make your baby follow your schedule instead.

Kevin, software engineer and father of Jacob, age 5 months
Texas

Focus on the baby's needs and your needs. It may seem like you will never get a routine down and your laundry is going to take over the house, but I promise as time goes on, you will figure out a routine that allows you to get all the housekeeping chores done effortlessly.

Jenny Lovins, professional organizer, author of *Unclutter Your Life*, and mother of Jacob, age 5, and Grace, age 2
Virginia

In my family, we tried to have our newborns fit into our schedule as much as we could so the pre-child difference would not be so shocking. It worked wonders!

Jamie Yasko-Mangum, certified image consultant and mother of Stone, age 4½, and Spencer, age 2½
Florida

STAY ON THE HOSPITAL SCHEDULE. Do not bring baby to bed and do not use any stimulus when putting baby(ies) to bed. This will keep them on a great sleeping schedule and start a good habit.

Nina, mother of Faith, age 10, and quadruplets Joseph, Nicole, John, and, Lynn, age 8
New York

Prior to having my son, a friend told me that the best thing her mother did for her while caring for her infant son was to put him down for a nap at 9 am – tired or not! Babies do take comfort in developing a sleeping and feeding schedule, so follow their lead!

Brenda, homemaker and mother of Kieran, 32 months
New Jersey

Bum/boobs/burp/bounce/bum/bed. On waking I found that if I followed this routine, it was really what babies need in the early days. Change them, feed them, burp them, play with them, possibly change them again, and ha! ha! Bed. Fortunately, my little one seemed to have read Gina Ford and fell in love with her ideas. Control the light in the sleeping area. You can cheat all summer with a blackout blind and still have tinies in bed by 7 pm. Hang onto the lunchtime nap for as long as possible. See it as a siesta – good food, good sleep, and good play equals a happy baby and sane parents.

Cath Shipton, TV actress and mother of Tallulah, age 3½
London, England

I believe that schedules are important in raising children to a certain degree. Sometimes you have to just go with the flow and let them take the lead for awhile. It will help to relax both you and your children. Control is only effective when you know how to give them control and when you know how to act with control.

Janell, mother of Morgan, age 8, and Emma, age 1
Pennsylvania

As soon as possible, get your baby on a schedule for napping, meals, and bedtime. By having a schedule, I can pretty much determine my baby's needs and prevent crying spells. As an example, my baby's lunch time is 11:30 am and nap time is 12:00 noon. If by noon I have not yet fed my little one and he begins to cry, I will know instantly what is bothering him. No more trying to figure out why he's upset. Also, with a schedule, it makes it a lot easier to plan my day with my baby, or my own free time and time with my husband.

Glenda, homemaker, business owner, and mother of
Sean, age 6, and Christian, age 2
California

It is most important and so helpful to get your child on a regular schedule. It makes for a happier baby and mom!

Beth, administrative assistant and mother of
Sarah Elizabeth, age 4, and Caroline Lillian, age 11 months
Delaware

Many parents say feed the baby when he's hungry; let the baby sleep when he's sleepy. That sounds good, but it is not practical. If you're feeding "whenever," how do you know how much and how often he needs to eat, and how will you learn to differentiate between cries? For new moms who are frazzled by all the demands on them, routines and schedules are very helpful. It's not to say they're not flexible. After all, your baby is a human, not a robot. One routine that helped both my sons sleep through the night was to keep them up after their 7 or 8 pm feeding by playing with them, walking around with them, or just putting them in their bouncy chair. I would then give them a nice, warm bath. After putting on their pajama's, I would shut off all the lights, lower the TV, and give them their last feeding. When they would wake up for night feedings, I would resist the temptation to interact with them and just feed them and rock them back to sleep. This worked for my 5-year-old. He slept through the night by 3 months, and my newborn is only 2 months and is sleeping through the night already!

Jocelyn, teacher and mother of Brandon, age 5, and Benjamin, age 2 months

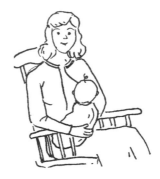

Breastfeeding Basics

When first nursing, be sure baby is in a straight line from tip to toes, facing your breast. If the head is turned to the side, there will be a twist in the throat, making it impossible to swallow milk.

Jacquie, mother of Alicia, age 16
Maryland

Make sure your baby is sucking squarely and securely on the entire nipple. Sucking on only a portion will inflame the area being sucked, making it extremely painful. I learned this the hard way. My baby got a firm grip on only one side of each nipple, and a crescent shaped area on each became swollen in the same manner as inflamed taste buds, only my baby wasn't sucking for dear life (every two hours) on my tongue! Nursing became an act of sheer will and pure, determined love because it hurt beyond belief. And don't make the mistake of thinking this could happen only with the innocence of breastfeeding for the first time. I had it happen with my second child as well.

Judith, English teacher and mother of Eugene, age 27, and Nina, age 26
Washington

Unwrap your newborn from the swaddling to nurse. It is so difficult to position baby correctly when he/she is so far away from your body.

Tammarra, mother of Bryden, age 8, and Ava, age 3
New York

When burping your baby, turn his/her head to the side. Your baby won't spit up as much.

Cathy , nurse and mother of Niki, age 3, Marina, age 1, and Baby # 3 due in April
New Jersey

Learn how to nurse your newborn lying down. Even if you are told that your little one can't do it until he's bigger, work at it anyway. Once you get him used to nursing while you lie down, you can get him to latch on and go back to sleep. It is a lifesaver those first few months when the baby nurses every couple of hours.

Brandy, professional birth assistant and mother
Colorado

There is an over-the-counter product called Lansinoh. It is pure lanolin and has wonderful qualities, including healing sore, cracked nipples. Buy a huge tube and use it beyond your breastfeeding days as it works miracles on chapped lips, too.

Meredith, marketing consultant and mother of Eliza, age 3, and Zachary, age 1½
New Jersey

The pillow called Breast Friend and the soft silicon nipple shield were my best companions when nursing! Also, for engorged breasts, use cabbage leaves. They are amazingly soothing!

Aggie, teacher and mother of Alexandra, age 2½, and Cassandra, 6 months
California

This tip from my son's first pediatrician, who had breastfed her own four children, probably saved our breastfeeding relationship right from the beginning. She told me, "Don't make breastfeeding an academic exercise. Throw away your watch! If your baby acts like he wants to nurse, don't worry about how long it's been since the last feeding – just go ahead and nurse him! You can't overfeed a breastfed baby." That mind-set has been essential with both of my children in establishing not only my milk supply to match their needs but also in helping us learn to communicate with one another from the earliest days. Eventually, with each child, we found a rhythm that worked for both of us.

Hannah, mother of Ian, age 4, and Eliza, age 13 months
South Carolina

I think mothers would greatly benefit from learning about their options with nursing sleepwear. Most nursing sleepwear out there are tent-style nightgowns with slits in the front to nurse through. Not only are these unfeasible for nursing, they are unattractive, and they do not help with holding in nursing pads. Mothers must wear a nursing bra under their nightgown, which adds to the uncomfortable issue and prolongs the time it takes to start nursing due to fiddling with their bra and then their nightgown. Look for nursing gowns that are comfortable, attractive, and help with nighttime nursing. They should hold nursing pads in place, have microelastic sewn in for support under the breasts, are made of a cotton/lycra blend for stretch, and have a split front design for quick access to the breast.

I think most new moms don't know what options they have.

Aimee Kendall, registered nurse, founder www.aimeegowns.com, and mother of Jacob, age 4, and Kolson, age 2

A friend of mine was frustrated with where to put her shirt when she breastfed. "I hadn't really thought about that," I said. "I just tuck it under my arm."

Kim, mother of Connor, age 3, and Heather, age 6 months

One of my favorite ways to breastfeed is lying down in bed. It is so comfortable for both mother and baby. But often my breast would leak milk, or my baby would spit up on my sheets and comforter. The last thing any mother wants is another load of laundry! My tip is to have a dozen old-fashioned cotton diapers folded by the bed – you just grab one and lay it flat under your breast and baby to catch any spilled milk. It is much easier to throw it in the hamper to wash!

Candace, The Bradley Method Childbirth Educator and stay-at-home mother of Perry Elizabeth, age 5, and Zoe Adair, age 18 months
Texas

Breastfeeding targets fat stores kept in a woman's thighs and behind, so it's one of the only times that you can easily reduce your fat in these areas without dieting or working out – yet another good reason to breastfeed your precious child. If you use lanolin for your chapped nipples when you're breastfeeding, you can wipe the excess off your fingers onto your dry lips. It works great as a chapstick!

Heidi, courtesy of The Center for Conscious Parenting, www.cfcp.info, "run-outside-of-the-house" mom and mother of Heather, age 20 months
Oregon

You will be gaining your confidence about a lot of things in the first days and weeks, and you'll be feeling particularly vulnerable to the comments of those around you. Encouraging words feel like a lifeline, and critiques stab at your heart. Because a lot of knowledge about breastfeeding was lost when formula was heavily marketed, your parents might not know much, if anything, about breastfeeding. Or perhaps your mother tried to breastfeed and was successful even, but her information could be dated. In any case, you might want to protect yourself from folks whose words or actions might undermine your confidence. If there is someone in your life who you will be counting on for support, invite him/her to be present during a doula shift or a visit with your lactation consultant. It will give them an opportunity to learn how to support you with breastfeeding (how to check the latch, position pillows, etc.), ask questions, and alleviate any concerns they have.

Karen Laing, lactation consultant, owner of Birthways Doula Services in Chicago, and mother of Birkleigh, age 9 months
Illinois

If your baby is having trouble latching on, try sticking your pinkie, fingernail-side down, into his/her mouth almost far back enough to gag him/her (but, of course, not quite that far). Do this right before latching him/her on to train his/her mouth to feel where the nipple should go. (This saved my sanity AND my nipples!)

Nancy Peske, writer and mother of Dante, age 5
New York

If your newborn's suck is not strong enough or he/she seems to be biting down on the breast with his/her gums, gently apply a little upward pressure to the lower chin bone as your baby sucks. It will help you child position his/her tongue better and provide a more efficient suck. This is also useful for babies having trouble with bottles.

Diane, labor and postpartum doula

Get comfortable with nursing while lying down. It makes a world of difference on the amount of sleep both you and your new baby will get at night.

Candice, doula and mother of Skyler, age 5½, Sylvia, age 3, and Sage, age 1
California

Practice breastfeeding while lying down during the daytime so you and your baby get the hang of it quickly while you can see what you're doing. Then you'll be able to get baby latched on quickly in the night and go back to sleep all the sooner!

Sharon, stay-at-home mother of William, age 7, and Stephen, age 5
Illinois

Instead of buying expensive breast pads, buy a pack of cheap sanitary towels. They do a better job and save lots of money.

Elizabeth, nursery nurse and mother of Rowan (as in tree), age 13 weeks

When in doubt, always offer the breast as a first option.

Jo-Anne, mother of seven, stepmother of two, and step-nanny of
four living and two angels
Canada

Crying can be a late sign of hunger! Babies let you know when they want to nurse by tongue "darting" (sticking their tongues in and out) and "rooting" (turning their heads side to side). Being watchful for these two things, as well as your child's own unique sounds or facial expressions, will give you the opportunity to respond to baby's need to nurse without having your child reach the point of crying.

Breast milk digests in a baby's stomach in only twenty minutes, because a baby's stomach is the size of a walnut, and breast milk is made for babies so it digests well. So, a baby can want to nurse more than once an hour and truly be hungry. All babies have their own rhythm of nursing, which also varies from day to day and over time. The best way to determine how much and when to nurse is when the baby indicates it's time.

Sherri , mother of Emma, age 3½
New York

It's tough in the beginning, but when you're feeding your baby while you are sleeping, you'll realize it's the greatest invention God ever came up with!

Amanda, stay-at-home mother of Samantha Alexis, age 11 months
Ohio

Remember, it is never possible to force a baby to breastfeed. If baby is hungry, he/she will nurse, and if not, he/she won't. Always try the breast first for a fussy baby – a baby's eating patterns are so unpredictable that chances are, if your child is fussy, he/she is probably hungry!

**Elizabeth, part-time seamstress and full-time mother of
Erin, age 13, Kelly, age 10, Drew, age 7, and Caitlin, age 5
Massachusetts**

Sharing your bed with your baby ensures a minimal amount of disruption at night and aids breastfeeding. My tip for this period in your life is to get rid of the clock in your bedroom so that you are not tempted to count or time your child's nursings. Treasure these moments snuggling your baby — they soon will be past!

**Barbara, mother of Felix, age 6, and Edgar, age 2
Yorkshire, United Kingdom**

Try not to create a "snacker." Feeding on demand does not mean that every time a baby cries he/she wants to eat. It is so important to have a "complete feed." That means as much as possible, you should stimulate and keep your baby feeding so that she doesn't eat for five minutes at a time and fall asleep. You may have to take off clothing, rub the bottom of her feet, change her diaper in mid-feed to reawake her. But with a full meal, she will be more satisfied and sleep more soundly, and you will get a much needed break! Also, during the first six weeks or so, a baby's awake cycle is only 45 to 60 minutes long. Baby wakes to eat, burp, be changed, and have a small window to interact. Then she is ready to be tightly swaddled and put back to sleep and should sleep for about 1½ to 2 hours. If you keep a baby up too long, he/she is easily overtired and has a hard time getting to sleep.

**Diane, labor/postpartum doula
Maryland**

Don't rely on the clock to feed your baby. Look for cues from the baby and go from that. This is the best way to satisfy your baby's needs and have a happy baby!

**Jennifer, certified childbirth educator and mother of
Amanda, age 5½, and Abby, age 2½
Georgia**

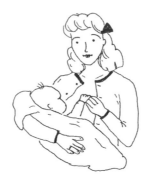

‑Nursing All the Time?‑

Don't forget the growth spurts! Many moms give up on nursing when their babies all of a sudden start wanting to nurse all the time and fussing in between feedings. More than likely these are the growth spurts the baby goes through, and the increased nursing signals to mom's body to produce more milk. Just hang in there and things will calm down in a few days.

Amy, homemaker and mother of
Joshua, age 6, Jesse, age 4, Grace, age 2, and another on the way
South Carolina

Patience, patience, patience is key. Babies, especially newborns, go through growth spurts just about the time that you are starting to get used to breastfeeding, and first time moms tend to worry what they are doing is wrong and if the baby is getting enough milk. Don't worry! It usually takes your breasts about a day to catch up to your baby's increase in appetite, and that first day of a growth spurt seems like you are constantly feeding. But be patient and ride through it and feed the baby as much as he/she wants. By the next day usually things calm down again to his/her regular 2 to 3 hour feeding pattern. Make sure you rest and drink lots of fluids, too!

Shaana, doula and CBE and mother of
Nicholaus, age 20 months, and expecting Baby #2 in March 2005
California

Babies eat often when first born. This does not mean you are not producing enough milk. It just means babies eat often when first born. Here are some tips. Keep baby close at night so you don't have to get up out of bed to feed your baby. And if you side lie, you can feed your baby while resting and not fully awake. Just remember to burp your baby so he/she won't wake up with a belly ache. No supplementation is usually necessary. Don't call your pediatrician or OB to find out if you are breastfeeding correctly: call a lactation consultant or a La Leche League leader. The lactation consultant will know lots more regarding breastfeeding questions and real problems.

Theresa, birth and postpartum doula and lactation counselor and mother of Jennifer, age 28, Erica, age 27, Michael, age 24, and Matthew, age 21
Connecticut

One of the most common concerns with new moms is wondering if you'll have enough breast milk to satisfy your baby. It's estimated that only about 2% of women truly cannot breastfeed or produce enough milk due to a medical condition. As for the others, it all works on supply and demand. The more you nurse your baby, the more milk you will produce. Your breasts are never empty. By introducing bottles and artificial baby milk, you are only sending signals to your body that it needs to make less milk. In the beginning weeks, it may feel like you are nursing nonstop. Since breast milk is more easily digested than formula, breastfed babies need to eat more frequently than formula fed babies; and you may very well be feeding your baby every 1 to 2 hours. It's also possible that your baby may want to nurse for 20 to 30 minutes per side or longer. Eventually, your baby will become more efficient at nursing and will be able to get more out in less amount of time. Just follow your baby's cues and feed on demand. Don't watch the clock or create a schedule, and you will surely have a successful breastfeeding relationship. Occasionally, your baby will go through growth spurts and have a need to nurse more often. During this time, it is not necessary to supplement, and it is actually discouraged. Your baby will do all the work to increase your supply and will not starve in the interim. Breastfeeding does not always come naturally for everyone, so if you are having difficulty, find an experienced mom to help you. There's nothing worse than going to relatives or doctors that have little or no experience with breastfeeding. With a good support system, you will surely be successful, and the rewards are priceless. The bond that breastfeeding creates is so incredible, and you will feel good about giving your baby the absolute best.

Deana, mother of Kadyn, age 10, Abrien, age 8, Jaena, age 5, Madalyn, age 3, and Jason, age 6 months
Ohio

If someone, even your doctor, tells you that you need to wean your baby in order to take a particular medication, double check first! Many medications are, in fact, compatible with breastfeeding or a similar medication can be found that is. La Leche League or a lactation consultant can double check for you and potentially save both you and your baby a lot of grief!

Mara, La Leche League leader, counselor when employed,
and stay-at-home mother of Gabrielle, age 4, and Alexander, age 1
Georgia

There will be days when the couch and TV will be your best friends. Find a comfy spot and let baby nurse for hours on end as he/she grows before your very eyes. You'll often question your ability to breastfeed and supply your baby with what he/she needs, but you can do it! It's a supply and demand relationship. Let your baby nurse and nurse and nurse for as long as it takes. The growth spurt will soon be over, and you will be more confident in your abilities to fulfill your baby's needs. Do not give in to temptation and think that formula will help! It won't. It breaks the supply and demand cycle and often is the culprit for a failed breastfeeding relationship.

Amanda, stay-at-home mother of Samantha Alexis, age 11 months
Ohio

It is important to breastfeed your newborn on demand. Unlike bottle-fed babies who eat every four to six hours, breastfed babies need to eat at least every two hours around the clock. (Breast milk digests quickly!) They will need to nurse even more frequently during growth spurts. To help prevent sore nipples, be sure your baby is latched on correctly; they should have most of the areola in their mouth. The best thing for sore nipples: lanolin cream.

Tanya, stay-at-home mother of Dennis, age 5, and Joseph, age 1
Florida

Don't give up during the first months when baby wants to eat "all the time" and the going is rough. The most enjoyable part of nursing and bonding is after the first six months. I wouldn't trade months 6 to 13 of breastfeeding my son for anything!

Vay, missionary and mother of Vinny
Indiana

Breastfeed early and often, even if it's only been a short time since the last nursing session. Babies often nurse at unpredictable intervals.

Liesl, professor of chemistry and mother of Liam, age 8 months
New Jersey

Throw the feeding schedule out the window and go with your baby's cues. Adults don't eat at the same time every day and the same amounts, so neither will babies. Their tummies are so tiny! Sometimes they will eat every half hour when going through a growth spurt.

Amanda, stay-at-home mother of Samantha Alexis, age 11 months
Ohio

If you have problems nursing (i.e., your baby is not gaining weight – a situation which can make any new mom lose her mind!), ask your doctor about the following strategy: Nurse for as long as you and/or the baby want to (even if only five minutes at first), then supplement with breast milk or formula. There are several ways to supplement the baby that won't cause nipple confusion. "Finger Feeding" through a syringe worked great for me and my baby. (The SNS device I tried at first drove me so crazy — I almost gave up nursing altogether.) The syringe strategy enabled us to get some experience nursing, but then allowed me to relax and know that my baby would get the nourishment he needed from the supplementation. Once he gained the weight he needed, we transitioned to full-time nursing. Unless you really want to nurse your baby ALL the time, ask your lactation consultant about when and how to introduce the bottle, just in case you might want a "mommy's night out" at some point!

Sarah Zeldman, Life Balance coach – Balanced Woman Coaching,
www.Balanced-woman-coaching.com,
and mother of Yosef, age 3½, and Shanya, age 1
New York

I'm about to explode! Frozen cabbage leaves are soothing on engorged breasts.

Terese, infant sign instructor and mother of a girl, age 4½, and a boy, age 2
Alberta, Canada

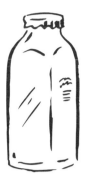

Pumping

If breastfeeding, give you and your baby time to get to know each other and your baby's feeding needs. I got advice from a maternity nurse to start pumping right away and take advantage of the surplus milk to save us in the freezer. It ended up being the worst decision I made. After my first session of expressing milk, I began to overproduce. My baby could not drain my breasts which led to blocked milk ducts and then mastitis. I had a fever of 103 and was in agony. It was miserable. I tell every new mom to wait before expressing milk. You and your baby need to get to know each other so you only produce as much as your baby needs. After about 6 weeks or so, then you can start to express for those moments when you need a break.

**Mary, sign language interpreter and mother of
Maura, age 2, and Rebecca, age 9 months
New Hampshire**

Invest in a decent pump. If possible, spend a little more for an electric one instead of the handheld versions. In the beginning, a pump can help if you become engorged. You can pump and store milk in your freezer in case of an emergency or if you need a night out. You can pump and dump if you decide to have the occasional glass of wine or extra latte.

**Barbara, former banker and mother of Jamie, age 4, and Kaleigh, age 1
Hawaii**

Women usually produce more milk in the morning and may have leftover milk after the first feeding of the day. This is an opportune time to "steal" a little milk by pumping and storing for later.

Heidi, courtesy of The Center for Conscious Parenting, www.cfcp.info, "run-outside-of-the-house" mom and mother of Heather, age 20 months Oregon

I recommend renting an "industrial" breast pump from the hospital. Although it looks like an escapee from the dairy farm, it really works quickly, allowing you to pump and store milk easily.

My son was born 12 weeks premature and had to stay in the hospital for almost eight weeks. I went home with a rented breast pump machine from the hospital and had to pump every three hours while he was in the hospital to maintain my supply. As a result I had a decent amount of stored milk when he came home.

I kept the industrial pump set up next to my bed and would continue to pump after the morning feedings or when someone was bottle feeding him and then store that milk. This way my husband, grandparents, or whoever wanted could feed Holden. I also bought a cheap pump to take if I was going to be working away from home for the day.

Feeding a baby is such an amazing bonding activity — whether it's from breast or bottle — and by regularly pumping and nursing, I was able to allow people who love my son to enjoy those wonderful bonding moments with him. I don't think I would have been able to feed my son breast milk for the whole first year if I was the only one doing it.

Connie, publisher and mother of Holden, age 3 New Jersey

While nursing my children, I pumped extra milk and donated it to Massachusetts General Hospital for preemies or babies born to addicted mothers. Not only did the extra pumping help me lose my pregnancy weight quickly, but I felt great helping others. After I was medically screened, the hospital provided everything: 2-ounce bottles and a UPS freezer pack which I sent in as soon as I had 60 bottles filled. I've since learned that this is done at hospitals all over the country. I lost those 50, yes 50, pregnancy pounds in record time.

Alison Ashley Formento, writer for harriedmom.com, and mother of Alex, age 7½, and Natalie, age 5 New Jersey

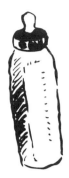

Bottle Feeding

I have a tip that saved me lots of time and energy. Because of my family's very busy lifestyle, I had to come up with something to make bottle making easier during the first 11 months of my daughter's life!! I decided early to wean my daughter from warm bottles to room temperature ones. The way I did this was I started giving her cooler and cooler bottles until I could use bottled water only and then used room temperature bottled water from then on. This made life a breeze!! Instead of always needing to mix formula with warm water, I could mix it with a bottle of bottled water anywhere at anytime!!! It was perfect. I also used the easy premeasured 8-ounce packs that are just rip, pour, add bottled water, shake, and away you go!! No worries about hot spots or anything!!! Just would like to pass this on to new moms finding out the hassles of warm bottles.

Coreen
Oregon

If you hand wash your bottles, breast pump, etc., get a pile of thin moist towelette washcloths. They're thin enough to reach into nipple tips and pump crevices – just thread them over the end of your bottle brush and wash away. They can also be bunched up thick enough to feel like a washcloth when washing inside bottles. I feel like I get large bottles that I can't reach into cleaner when I wrap one of these thin washcloths around the brush and then use that to wipe the inside of the bottle.

Laureen, teacher and mother of Jacob, age 5 months
Texas

I ended up back in the hospital, via the emergency room, the day I went home with my baby and was diagnosed with acute eclampsia/toxemia. Therefore, all my plans for breastfeeding went down the drain! I beat myself up for it and felt guilty, thinking that my baby wouldn't be as healthy growing up as a breastfed baby (as I had read and my doctor had told me). Now my daughter is a very healthy grown woman of 21 years. She never had anything other than your occasional common cold. Do not feel guilty if things don't go as you had planned. Your baby will be fine!

Trisha, senior executive assistant and mother of Erica Nicole, age 21
California

When burping your baby, turn his/her head to the side. Your baby won't spit up as much.

Cathy, nurse and mother of Niki, age 3, Marina, age 1, and Baby # 3 due in April
New Jersey

For some women breastfeeding does not come easy and can be painful as well as frustrating. I was grateful to learn that I was not the only woman to experience a variety of issues. Although I would have wanted to breastfeed longer then I did (three months), Mother Nature had other plans for me. My child is now 7 and doing wonderful despite the short time we breastfed.

Laurie Bagley, Owner of Fit Maternity & Beyond and mom to Avriel, age 7
California

Buy powdered formula and mix it with warm water, as needed. No need to heat the bottle or keep it cool while traveling. I always kept some bottled water in the car so we could easily make a room-temperature bottle on the go!

Meredith, marketing consultant and mother of Eliza, age 3, and Zachary, age 1½
New Jersey

My preemie was a poor eater. I would mix his jar food in with his formula and cut a little x in the nipple so the thicker formula would flow free. This would make me feel better that I was able to get more food into him.

Charlotte Du Brier, author of *How Not to be a Frazzled Bride*
and mother of Marc David
Pennsylvania

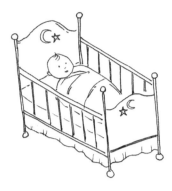

Newborn Sleep

A lot of parents worry about moving around and doing things quietly so the baby gets good rest. Gosh knows, no one wants to be in charge of a child who didn't get the full rest he/she needed. My tip: make lots of noise during the day and keep the room bright. Vacuum by their faces – do anything you would normally need to do and do it with the baby close by. My children can sleep through a train wreck now, and I owe it all to dishes, CNN news, and the lovely people from Oreck!

Jennifer, stay-at-home wife and mother of Magolia, age 4, and Van Royal, age 2
Utah

Even with Baby #1, don't be afraid to do things while the baby is sleeping (assuming you're like me and ignored the other advice to nap when your baby naps). The more you can get your new baby acclimated to the truly normal noises of the household, the better. He/She will be able to go to and stay asleep much better on his/her own if not "protected" from the noise. So be it a dog barking to be let in, a phone conversation with a friend, or my all-time favorite, the vacuum, let it go (within reason). If you spend all your time tip-toeing around and hushing everyone, you're only setting yourself up for many days and nights of disturbed sleep for you and baby.

Marie, human resources director and mother of
Paul, age 12, and Jane, age 10
New Jersey

Don't feel the need to turn off the ringer, post notes on your door to not ring the doorbell, etc., when your baby is sleeping. Most babies are not bothered by such details. It is better to condition them to sleep through "noise" so that they don't become accustomed to absolute silence which will be problematic in the future when you can't control the noise level.

Christie, project director for a graphic design firm and mother of Jackson, age 4, and Mackenzie, age 5 months
New Jersey

When my second child was born, she would always wake up the minute I put her down in her bed, no matter how hard I tried to do it as smoothly as possible. One day, for some reason, I decided to wrap up a heating pad in a baby blanket and place it on medium in her bassinet. When the time came to lay her down, I removed the heating pad and laid her down. To my complete delight, she didn't wake up. My advice is don't let a warm cheek touch a cold sheet.

Ronica, doula and mother of Katherine, age 11, Rachael, age 6, and BJ, age 5
Oregon

It is very natural for a newborn to fall asleep while sucking at the breast, a bottle, or a pacifier. When a baby always falls asleep this way, he learns to associate sucking with falling asleep; over time, he cannot fall asleep any other way. I have heard a number of sleep experts refer to this as a "negative sleep association." I certainly disagree, and so would my baby. It is probably the most positive, natural, pleasant sleep association a baby can have. However, a large percentage of parents who are struggling with older babies who cannot fall asleep or stay asleep are fighting this natural and powerful sucking-to-sleep association.

Therefore, if you want your baby to be able to fall asleep without your help, it is essential that you sometimes let your newborn baby suck until he is sleepy, but not totally asleep. When you can, remove the breast, bottle, or pacifier from his mouth and let him finish falling asleep without something in his mouth. When you do this, your baby may resist, root, and fuss to regain the nipple. It's perfectly okay to give him back the breast, bottle, or pacifier and start over a few minutes later. If you do this often enough, he will eventually learn how to fall asleep without sucking.

Elizabeth Pantley, author of *The No-Cry Sleep Solution: Gentle Ways to Help Your Baby Sleep Through the Night* (Excerpted with permission by McGraw-Hill/ Contemporary Publishing. www.pantley.com/elizabeth) and mother of Angela, age 17, Vanessa, age 15, David, age 14, and Coleton, age 5
Washington

A newborn baby sleeps about sixteen to eighteen hours per day, and this sleep is distributed evenly over six to seven brief sleep periods. You can help your baby distinguish between nighttime sleep and daytime sleep and thus help him sleep longer periods at night.

Begin by having your baby take his daytime naps in a lit room where he can hear the noises of the day, perhaps a bassinet or cradle located in the main area of your home. Make nighttime sleep dark and quiet. You can also help your baby differentiate day naps from night sleep by using a nightly bath and a change into sleeping pajamas to signal the difference between the two.

One way to encourage good sleep is to get familiar with your baby's sleepy signals and put her down to sleep as soon as she seems tired. A baby cannot put herself to sleep, nor can she understand her own sleepy signs. Yet a baby who is encouraged to stay awake when her body is craving sleep is typically an unhappy baby. Over time, this pattern develops into sleep deprivation, which further complicates your baby's developing sleep maturity. Learn to read your baby's sleepy signs — such as quieting down, losing interest in people and toys, and fussing — and put her to bed when that window of opportunity presents itself.

Elizabeth Pantley, author of *The No-Cry Sleep Solution: Gentle Ways to Help Your Baby Sleep Through the Night* (Excerpted with permission by McGraw-Hill/ Contemporary Publishing. www.pantley.com/elizabeth) and mother of Angela, age 17, Vanessa, age 15, David, age 14, and Coleton, age 5 Washington

Teach your baby to fall asleep on his/her own. You can do this by putting him/her down while still awake or just about to fall asleep. This is a big time and energy saver for you as you won't need to rock or hold baby to sleep.

Kristi, technical support and mother of Ethan, age 5 months Washington

Rocking your baby is such a sweet time. After you have rocked the baby, be sure to lay your newborn down for nap/sleeptime while he/ she is still awake. The baby will learn to fall asleep on his/her own. This will help later on when it is time for the baby to sleep through the night.

Cherie Drennan, lighting designer, www.heavenly-lights.com, and mother of Johnny, age 12, Jordan, age 11, Olivia, age 9, Whit, age 7, and Gregory, age 3 Tennessee

Sure, waking up in the middle of the night with your baby can be exhausting. But think of it as special bonding time. Use only a night-light or flashlight to guide you. Keep talking at a minimum. Sit in a comfortable chair, such as a rocker, and feed your child. Don't stimulate or arouse your child with noise or excess light. Enjoy the quiet time together. And once she has been fed, burped, and changed (again, using minimal light – I kept a flashlight on the changing table!), place her in her crib/bassinet. Allow her to learn to self-calm. If she is fussy, let her know you are there by rubbing her back briefly or maybe placing her hand in her mouth. But don't resort to picking her up at the first sign of fussiness. Provide her with tools so that she alone can get herself to sleep. Try not to rely on music, rocking, car rides, holding, feeding, etc., to regularly get a child to go to sleep. It may take a little while, but your child (and you) will ultimately sleep better because of it!

Patricia, housewife, attorney, and mother of
Kaitlin, age 5, and Ashley, age 3½
New York

Don't forget that you are in charge when it comes to your newborn's sleep. After the first couple of weeks, don't be scared to put your baby to bed when he/she is tired. Keep an eye on the clock: every two hours your child is tuckered! Babies look for you to do this. It's comforting, and they realize sleep is a healthy pattern, not something you do when you are strung out. Wait a minute or two before you go in if you hear you child fuss (as long as it's not an urgent cry). They may have just rolled over and need a moment. Bottom line — take charge. We do it with what our children eat, play with, wear, etc…why not sleep? When you have a rested, happy child, you will be thankful for those times you clenched your fists and let them fuss for a minute.

Wendy, counselor and mother of Katie, age 14 months, and Baby #2 on the way
New Jersey

When you bring your child home from the hospital, don't tiptoe around your sweet bundle at naptime. Put his/her bassinet in a busy part of the house (den, living room). The baby will learn to sleep with background noises and do well under any circumstance. They say the womb is a loud place anyway.

Cherie Drennan, lighting designer, www.heavenly-lights.com, and mother of
Johnny, age 12, Jordan, age 11, Olivia, age 9, Whit, age 7, and Gregory, age 3
Tennessee

Always put newborns to bed awake so they will know how to fall asleep on their own (especially if they wake in the night!).

Paula Messner, musician and mother of Charlotte, age 6, and Rebecca, age 4
Missouri

From the first day home baby's room should be nice and light with the possibility of being pitch black when blinds, curtains, or shutters are closed. It is very important that when the baby goes down to sleep the room is very dark. This helps the baby define the difference between night and day and also helps to prevent the child from being scared of the dark when waking during the night. It is important that no shards of light come through the window as this is one of the most common problems with children waking very early in the morning. Also, if or when the baby wakes in the night, you want to try and get him/her used to drifting back off to sleep. But if shards of light escape through the room, it creates a huge distraction and keeps the baby awake.

Kelly, maternity nanny
Paris, France

Everyone will have an idea of how your baby should be sleeping, but ultimately your child will have his/her own developmental schedule for sleeping. Trust yourself and your baby, and trust that you will eventually sleep a full night again!

Lori, mother of Madeleine, age 9 months
Texas

Change your baby's outfit/pajamas before bedtime and when he/she wakes up in the morning. This helps babies get used to a nighttime and morning routine, which really helps when they are toddlers who resist getting their clothes changed at all!

Glynis, stay-at-home mother of Ryan, age 2
Georgia

Especially at night, the swaddle is so successful in getting the baby back to sleep. It is all about sleep deprivation when you have a newborn.

Georgeanne, labor and postpartum doula and mother of
four and grandmother of four
Maryland

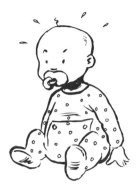

Sleeping All Night

During the early months of your baby's life, he sleeps when he is tired, it's really that simple. You can do very little to force a new baby to sleep when he doesn't want to sleep, and conversely, you can do little to wake him up when he is sleeping soundly.

Elizabeth Pantley, author of *The No-Cry Sleep Solution: Gentle Ways to Help Your Baby Sleep Through the Night* (Excerpted with permission by McGraw-Hill/ Contemporary Publishing. www.pantley.com/elizabeth) and mother of Angela, age 17, Vanessa, age 15, David, age 14, and Coleton, age 5
Washington

As a new mom, it was really hard to hear my baby cry and not go in and pick him up. But, as a single mom, I also had to work and needed my own sleep to do that. What really helped me was something I learned from Penelope Leach in her book *Your Baby and Child*. If my baby started crying in the middle of the night, I would go in and determine if he was okay. Then I would comfort him with a few soothing words and a rub on the back. Then I would leave, set a timer for 15 minutes and fall back to sleep. If he was still crying when the timer went off, I would go back and do the same thing again. He soon learned that mom was nearby and would comfort him but wouldn't take him out of bed. This helped me feel like I was responding to his need for comfort without disrupting my whole night. It was essential to our successfully navigating those early months.

Lynne, social work administrator and mother of Brint, age 18
Alabama

A very important point to understand about newborn babies is that they have very, very tiny tummies. New babies grow rapidly, their diet is liquid, and it digests quickly. Formula digests quickly and breast milk digests even more rapidly. Although it would be nice to lay your little bundle down at a predetermined bedtime and not hear a peep from him until morning, even the most naïve among us know that this is not a realistic goal for a tiny baby. Newborns need to be fed every two to four hours — and sometimes more.

During those early months, your baby will have tremendous growth spurts that affect not only daytime, but also nighttime feeding as well, sometimes pushing that two- to four-hour schedule to a one- to two-hour schedule around the clock. Many pediatricians recommend that parents shouldn't let a newborn sleep longer than three or four hours without feeding, and the vast majority of babies wake far more frequently than that. (There are a few exceptional babies who can go longer.) No matter what, your baby will wake up during the night. The key is to learn when you should pick her up for a night feeding and when you can let her go back to sleep on her own.

This is a time when you need to focus your instincts and intuition. This is when you should try very hard to learn how to read your baby's signals. Here's a tip that is critically important for you to know.

Babies make many sleeping sounds, from grunts to whimpers to outright cries, and these noises don't always signal awakening. These are what I call sleeping noises, and your baby is nearly or even totally asleep during these episodes. I remember when my first baby, Angela, was a newborn. Her cry awakened me many times, yet she was asleep in my arms before I even made it from cradle to rocking chair. She was making sleeping noises. In my desire to respond to my baby's every cry, I actually taught her to wake up more often!

You need to listen and watch your baby carefully. Learn to differentiate between these sleeping sounds and awake and hungry sounds. If she is awake and hungry, you'll want to feed her as quickly as possible. If you respond immediately when she is hungry, she will most likely go back to sleep quickly. But, if you let her cry escalate, she will wake herself up totally, and it will be harder and take longer for her to go back to sleep. Not to mention that you will then be wide awake, too!

Elizabeth Pantley, author of *The No-Cry Sleep Solution: Gentle Ways to Help Your Baby Sleep Through the Night* (Excerpted with permission by McGraw-Hill/ Contemporary Publishing. www.pantley.com/elizabeth) and mother of Angela, age 17, Vanessa, age 15, David, age 14, and Coleton, age 5 Washington

My friends think I'm crazy or that I've really caught onto something good here. Both of my boys, Matthew, age 4, and Ryan, age 2, began sleeping through the night within their first six weeks of life – what a relief! Their pediatrician (who is wonderful) explained to me that sleeping is not just a natural behavior but a learned behavior. Just as we (well, most of us) don't wake up every few hours for something to eat, babies need to be weaned from this behavior and learn to comfort themselves and sleep through the night. Likewise, the process of falling asleep is a learned behavior. A routine – whatever works for you and your schedule — is so, so important. My boys genuinely learned when it was time to go to sleep through our evening rituals. Once more, it was important to put them to sleep while they were still awake so that they would learn to comfort themselves and fall asleep on their own. Again, putting yourself to sleep is a learned behavior at bedtime and throughout the night. I don't know about you, but my mom doesn't come over at 3 a.m. to rock me back to sleep when I wake up stressed about bills! Again, a learned behavior. My tip is not for the weak at heart; and trust me it wasn't easy. As my boys were adjusting to a schedule, I began to let those periods between waking up in the middle of the night lengthen before rushing to comfort them — two minutes one night, five minutes the next, and so on. Listening to your baby cry for a minute, much less five, is just torture, but there is a payoff. I would peek in, make sure everything was okay, change a diaper if needed, and just pat my baby's back for a minute. As the nights progressed, the length of time I waited grew and the time it took for them to fall back asleep shortened until they were sleeping through the night, and so was I! Payoff! They've learned that their bed is a place of comfort and security. Richard Ferber, M.D., wrote a much more scientific and detailed book on the subject titled *Solve Your Child's Sleep Problems*. What's great about this book is that Dr. Ferber offers methods which can be used for all young ages as well as various sleep problems. It's really fascinating. Those five minutes I would wait before going into my son's room to console him seemed like an eternity. But now I have such a peace of mind (and get much needed sleep after a busy day chasing those two monkeys!) when I put my boys to bed and know they are resting peacefully until the sun comes up.

Raquel , mother of Matthew, age 4, and Ryan, age 2
New Jersey

To sometimes help a child sleep through the night, you may want to give him/her a blanket or lovey. When choosing a lovey, the best kinds to try first should have satin. To help ease it into the baby/ toddler's life, try sleeping with it yourself for a few days, then give it to your child. The satin will naturally pick up your mommy-smell, and your child will be comforted when going to sleep with his/her new lovey or blanket since the scent of Mommy will be there.

Kathryn Peddle, owner/creator of Buddy Blankies and mother of
Robyn, age 7, and Richard, age 3
Canada

Both of my children were sleeping through the night by 8 weeks old. My "trick" was a few things combined: 1. no lights on 2. no talking 3. move fast and 4. biggest feeding last.

My goal was an 11 p.m. bedtime in the newborn days and a 6 a.m. or later wakeup hour. With my own babies, speed was the key part. The faster I arrived to a cry, the less agitated they got and the easier they went back down to sleep. The less time the babies spent awake, the less likely they were to get used to a feeding at that hour and ultimately didn't need to be fed or changed during the night.

Jennifer, stay-at-home wife and mother of Magolia, age 4, and Van Royal, age 2
Utah

Add a little rice cereal to the milk bottle before bedtime. Rice cereal is easy on the digestive tract.

Melanie, full-time domestic engineer, educator, author, and mother of twins
Meldonár and Meldoníque
Massachusetts

You have probably heard that babies should start "sleeping through the night" at about two to four months of age. What you must understand is that, for a new baby, a five-hour stretch is a full night. Many (but nowhere near all) babies at this age can sleep uninterrupted from midnight to 5 a.m. (Not that they always do.) A far cry from what you may have thought "sleeping through the night" meant!

What's more, while the scientific definition of "sleeping through the night" is five hours, most of us wouldn't consider that anywhere near a full night's sleep for ourselves. Also, some of these sleep-through-the-nighters will suddenly begin waking more frequently, and it's often a full year or even two until your little one will settle into a mature, all-night, every night sleep pattern.

Elizabeth Pantley, author of *The No-Cry Sleep Solution: Gentle Ways to Help Your Baby Sleep Through the Night* (Excerpted with permission by McGraw-Hill/ Contemporary Publishing. www.pantley.com/elizabeth) and mother of Angela, age 17, Vanessa, age 15, David, age 14, and Coleton, age 5
Washington

Sleeping through the night doesn't really mean what it says! Five hours is considered sleeping through the night by the American Academy of Pediatrics. Even now at 11 months, my baby still doesn't do that, but we have survived. So can you!

Amanda, stay-at-home mother of Samantha Alexis, age 11 months
Ohio

I am a mother of four children. The last children I had are identical twin girls. I learned a lot after my first two. I was losing lots of sleep and not getting any rest with them. I read books and found an article about how to get your baby to sleep all night. It was a great one, and it paid off big time. It said never put your baby in the bed with you. Your baby will get used to being in the bed with parents, and it will be extremely hard to get him/her to sleep in his/her own bed when the time comes. Another point was always feed your baby and change his/her diaper before bedtime, make sure the baby is going to be okay, and always put your baby on his/her back, never face down. Leave the room and check on baby throughout the night. I used a baby monitor beside my bed so if I heard something, I would check on my baby. If one of my twins cried, I would go ahead and feed her and change her diaper. I would then wake the other twin up and feed her. Actually, I fed them at the same time. I did this for about two weeks, and they were sleeping all night at 2½ months. I was blessed with two good twins, and I got my rest, and it was wonderful.

Beverly, mother of twins Brittany and Tiffany, age 4
Virginia

Okay – one thing I repeat over and over to my friends who are pregnant...your child can sleep through the night sooner than you probably expect and sooner than most parents allow. I truly believe a great deal of it is in the parents' control. Granted, we probably got very lucky with our first — she slept through the night at 5 weeks and virtually has not woken up again since. My tip is that once your child shows you that he/she can sleep an extended period of time — even if it isn't through the whole night — then help your child stick to that. Babies have their own little alarm clocks, and, of course, they would prefer a breast or bottle if they know they get it every time they cry. After two months of sleeping through the night our daughter woke up at 3 a.m. crying. I was so shocked I ran in and immediately nursed her. Of course, the next night, like clock work, she woke up at 3 a.m. I again nursed her. Then it occurred to me what was going on. The third night, when she woke up, I let her cry for a while. After twenty minutes I soothed her with my voice and hand but did not pick her up. After I left she cried for another twenty minutes. I did the same routine until she was asleep. This happened for two nights (they weren't fun) and never happened again. I feel confident that if I had continued to nurse her she would still wake up to this day at that time. I believe a lot of parents can prevent some of their sleeplessness and that, to a degree, babies are trainable in the sleep direction.

Michelle, courtesy of The Center for Conscious Parenting, www.cfcp.info,
stay-at-home-mother of Aidan, age 2
Oregon

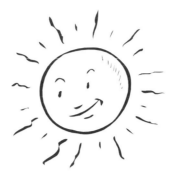

Napping

Most babies less than a year old have a three to three-and-a-half hour threshold before they get really cranky. Most of the time, it's because they're tired. Never underestimate the power of a good nap. Give your baby one nap in the morning and one nap in the afternoon at consistent times each day. Your baby will be happier and refreshed, and you will get a chance to get some things done around the house or catch up on a few winks yourself.

Maria Garcia, owner Get Organized Now! and mother of Amanda, age 7 months Wisconsin

One thing that I always did with my babies was to make a real difference between daytime sleeping and nighttime sleeping. When they were sleeping during the day, I would put them in a different room or a different place than they slept in at night. I would also not make it very quiet but go about whatever I was doing, as well I wouldn't make it dark. Then when it was time to sleep at night they would be in their crib, and it would be dark and quiet. Another thing I found helpful in getting them to sleep through the night was to be very quick and efficient with whatever had to be done when they woke up in the night.

Courtesy of the moms of Blackberry Creek Community Church in Aurora, IL

Never, ever wake a sleeping baby.

Daniela "Skittles" Burckhardt, singer of the CandyBand

Here is a good way to teach your newborn that nighttime is for sleep and daytime is for fun. If the baby wakes up hungry or needs a diaper change and it is nighttime, then do what you need to in as little light as possible. Do not play with the baby or make any noise (babbling, singing, etc.). Basically, make nighttime boring. If the baby is crying and needs to be comforted, then by all means pick him/her up and give comfort. But keep the TV off and stay away from the computer or any other distraction. During the day, put the baby to nap in a place that has more light and noise than the nighttime situation. This is a good gentle way to help a baby learn that nighttime is for sleeping. It is not traumatic like putting a child in another room and ignoring their cries.

Candice, doula and mother of Skyler, age 5½, Sylvia, age 3, and Sage, age 1
California

I swaddle my baby, even at 4 months old, at nap time because it makes him feel secure and cozy. When I started doing this, he went from taking short 20- or 30-minute catnaps to 2-hour naps during the day. Another important tip is to always put your baby down for naps while he is still awake. This way he learns to put himself to sleep. If he awakens at some point during the nap, he will know how to fall back asleep on his own.

Jessica, public relations and mother of Kane, age 4 months
Tennessee

When putting your baby down for a nap, place his/her bed in a "high traffic" area (living room, kitchen), and do "loud" housework like vacuuming, dishes, etc. This trains your baby to differentiate between daytime sleep and nighttime sleep and also trains him/her to be a deep sleeper.

Darlene, home business entrepreneur and homeschooling mother of
Simon, age 11, and Christina, age 9½
Canada

When you are introducing a new routine to a baby, you should make sure that walks are taken during a nap time or baby will not be ready for his/her scheduled sleep afterwards. Taking baby for a walk during a scheduled nap allows him/her to have a good sleep; and when you arrive home, he/she will be hungry and ready for the next feeding. This fits in where it works. Usually the best time is in the afternoon after baby's feeding and before bath time.

Kelly, maternity nanny
Paris, France

— Better Bedtimes —

Originally, I was waiting to see what my daughter's own sleep schedule was, but after about a year, a friend recommended making a consistent 7 pm bedtime. We have found this to be a really positive thing for our whole family. I would have started it from the very beginning if I had known then what I know now.

Sherri, mother of Emma, age 3½
New York

To train your baby to understand a reasonable bedtime, try the following. After the first feeding after 6 pm, change your baby, put him into pajamas, and put him to bed. This creates a regular bedtime at a reasonable time in the evening, leaving you enough time to connect with your spouse/partner before your own bedtime. In the morning, you decide what time is a reasonable time to get up and treat any waking up before this time as you would a night waking. In other words, make sure your baby is fed and comfortable; then put him back to bed. He may fuss a bit, but you must remain firm and consistent. Doing this right from day one, both of my children (one of whom was colicky) learned to sleep from 7 pm to 7 am from a very early age. They are still excellent sleepers a decade later.

Darlene, home business entrepreneur and homeschooling mother of
Simon, age 11, and Christina, age 9½
Canada

Many moms I knew complained about how they couldn't get their baby to bed which I did not understand. My son, Steven, was adopted from Russia as an infant. As someone who had a baby that crossed 11 time zones, I was not only able to get him back on a regular sleep schedule, we were able to have a baby who went to bed (and still does to this day) without fussing or crying. I believe it was because we had not just created a routine, but we had designed a daily evening ritual that came to become a comfort for child and parents alike.

Every single NIGHT Steven got a bath. Yes, each and every night after dinner, I would bathe Steven, massage him with lotion, play about 10 minutes of Baby Mozart on videotape, and then I would sit and read to him for another few minutes in his room. Then we would cuddle for another five or ten minutes while listening to gentle, relaxing music. It was like a drill. And just like magic, my little one went to bed without fussing at all. He still does to this day, even to the extent of listening to the same CD he has listened to every night for the past five years! This little evening ritual has worked for friends' children who have stayed with us. Children need continuity, and the combination of these steps created a drowsy, relaxed child who was ready and willing to go to bed.

**Kathryn Weber, master Feng Shui consultant, publisher of *The Red Lotus Letter Feng Shui* e-zine (www.redlotusletter.com),
and mother of Angela, age 14, and Steven, age 5
Texas**

Always put your baby to bed awake. This teaches the baby to not rely on mommy or daddy to drift off into dreamland. Best advice the pediatrician ever gave us. All three of our children were sleeping through the night at a very early age.

**Lisa, director of quality and compliance and mother of
Evan Jacob, age 5, Emily Morgan, age 3, and Juliana Paige, 6 months
New Jersey**

To facilitate "story time" for my older son and to help my baby fall asleep without nursing, his dad takes him out to the hammock and swings him to sleep. It's been wonderful for all of us! No more crying at bedtime.

**Kelly, doula, president of the Albuquerque Birth Network,
and mother of two
New Mexico**

Start with the bedtime that you would ultimately like to have and make sure that you do your bedtime routine at that time from the beginning — even if you know the baby will only sleep 15 minutes — and make it EARLY!! This is my number one tip to new parents. We started with a 7:00 bedtime and at times we have put our kids to bed as early as 5:30. They will go and sleep through the night (not wake up at 5:30 to 6:00 am), contrary to what many moms think. This works better if you are home with your kids and really need to rely on an early bedtime every night to know that you have an end to your mommy day. It's also essential if you want to try and start a business. We started both of our kids on a bedtime routine at 10 days old. After dinner we have the bath. For bath I always suggest that you have warm water, lights off, lavender or some sort of soothing candles lit out of harms way, light music or soft sounds, and Epsom salt and lavender bubble bath. Sounds like a lot, but it really does soothe baby and signal that its time to relax. (Think of how that set up would make you melt?) Then breast/bottle feed by same candle light and light or soft sounds, and then lay down for bed. Even if you know the baby will wake up shortly, it starts to train baby's body to get that this is the time for bed.

Jennifer Fleece, owner/designer of Fleece Baby, www.fleecebaby.com, and mother of Killan, age 3 and Eloise, age 1½
Georgia

I am Mom to 5-year-old Emily and 16-month-old triplets Adam, Luke, and Julia. When Emily was born, I never wanted to let her cry herself to sleep. I had the time and the desire to rock her or nurse her to sleep every night. Unfortunately, to this day, she thinks she needs either my husband or me to fall asleep. She really resists going to bed on her own. So when the next three came along, I knew we had to do things differently…it would be impossible to rock all three of them to sleep. When the time came, we began putting them down in their cribs with their "blankies" while still awake so that they would learn to put themselves to sleep. For a few weeks, one, two, or all three of them would cry. We almost never went back into the room once they were put down. The duration of the crying lessened as time passed, and it didn't take long before they accepted both naps and bedtime with open arms. Many moms before me had urged me to do the same with Emily. I didn't listen to them then, but now my younger ones are testament to the fact that developing good sleeping habits for your baby depends a lot on your own courage and determination.

Lori, mother of Emily, age 5, and triplets Adam, Luke, and Julia, age 16 months

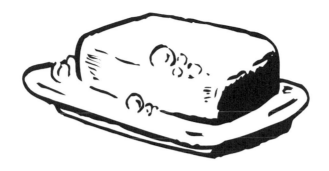

Bathing & Skin Care

My mother-in-law told me about putting Vaseline (nursery jelly) on my 6-week-old son's broken-out face/cheeks. It works like magic!

Lori, part-time pharmacy tech and full-time mother of Cale, age 2
Illinois

Don't try to clip a baby's fingernails with traditional clippers and risk clipping a finger with it. Just bite their nails instead. I know we've been taught not to bite our nails, but you don't risk hurting them. Their nails are thin, and if you bite them at one corner and just pull with your teeth, the rest of the nail pulls right off. I have two children and have never ripped a nail below the skin nor have I ever clipped a squirming finger. Besides, the baby finds it much more fun to have his/her fingers in mom's mouth than a little metal sharp thing coming at him/her. And when baby gets older, that shiny metal sharp thing is too interesting for baby not to touch. If you have to use clippers, do it while your child is sleeping. Although, for me, that woke my child up.

Diana, homemaker and mother of Logan, age 3, and Anika, age 3 months
New Jersey

After baby's daily bath or sponge bath, use a cotton ball to apply baby oil to all of baby's skin folds and crevices. You will never have a problem with dry skin or chaffing.

Marlyne, mother of two adult children
Wisconsin

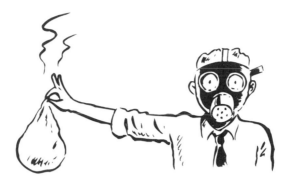

Diapers

Mothering a newborn is not about sweet puffs of baby powder and happy cooing. It's about poop, snot, and vomit: measuring it, worrying about it, wearing it, and cleaning it up. It's best to expect this so you are not disillusioned when you get your bundle of joy home.

Leigh Donadieu, publisher of *Cuizine* magazine and mother of Mitchell, age 4, and Ruth, age 2
New Jersey

When changing a little boy's diaper, use a washcloth to cover him when the diaper isn't on. I had to do this with my son, or we would both be soaked. It was well worth the added washcloths I washed.

Dawn, mother of Elizabeth, age 9, Tabitha, age 8, William, age 5, and Abigail, age 1
Virginia

A StrollerFit friend of mine had a great idea to keep her little one from squirming away while diaper changing. Use stickers to distract your baby by placing them on her arms and hands. She'll forget you're changing her diaper and play with the colorful stickers instead. Remove afterwards to avoid swallowing.

Kelly, fitness specialist and mother of Isabella, age 10 months
Texas

To keep little hands busy on the changing table, I put stickers on the backs of my baby's hands while changing her diaper. By the time she peeled them off, I had already completed changing her diaper.

Kristi, therapist and mother of Zoe, age 15 months
Texas

When I am changing my baby's diaper and he starts to cry, I try to remember to slow down rather than rush it and end up putting it on backwards. It helps to have patience.

Stephenie, homemaker and mother of Preston, age 3 months
Texas

It's time to move up to the next size diaper when your baby has had three consecutive poops that shoot up and out the top or sides of the diaper.

Ann Israel, Lamaze certified birth educator, certified prenatal yoga teacher, and mother of Ben, age 12, and Stephen, age 10
Maryland

When changing nappies (diapers), take a terry towel, fold it in half, place it on a changing mat with the short edge in line with the end of the changing mat, and place baby on top. The towel absorbs any "accidents" that can, and do, occur during nappy changes, and with the free end you can dab any areas that need dabbing.

Natasha, driving instructor and mother of identical twins, Sadie and Ruby, age 4
Hertfordshire, England

If you don't like the lingering smell of Desitin on your fingers, try saving the wrappers from nursing pads or other similar wrappers. I use Lansinoh pads and tear the outer wrapper in half, creating two mini envelopes just the right size to cover a finger when applying diaper rash ointment. Turn inside out after use, and you've never touched the stuff you just spread on your baby's bottom.

Laureen, teacher and mother of Jacob, age 5 months
Texas

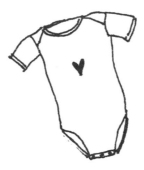

Dressing

My mother taught me this great laundry tip when my first son, Colin, was born. Fill a medium-size cleaning bucket with hot water and baby laundry detergent. Keep it in the bathroom, laundry room, or a place closest to where you change the baby. Every time you change an article of clothing (yours or the baby's) that has been spit up on, peed on, or soiled with formula or breast milk, toss it in the "soaking bucket." At the end of the day, pour out the water and toss the soaked clothing into the washing machine. This procedure really helps to remove difficult stains and keeps the baby laundry from piling up.

Monica, direct sales consultant and mother of Colin, age 8½
Texas

Connect the Velcro tabs of bibs before you put them in the wash, or you will be unsticking them from socks and everything else in the wash.

Allison, mother of Brindley, age 13 months
Texas

The best advice I ever got about dressing the baby and deciding if he would be warm enough came from my mom. She told me to always dress my baby in the same weight clothes I was wearing. "If mom is comfortable, baby will be comfortable." I thought about this a lot when I'd see babies in 100 degree weather wrapped in blankets and sleepers.

Linda, doula
Oklahoma

Any parent of an active baby has asked this question: "When should my child start wearing shoes?" There is no clear consensus. Some parents buy shoes as soon as their baby pulls herself into a first tentative stand; others wait as long as possible, preferring not to constrict their child's feet. As a general rule, kids will need shoes when they are ready to start walking around outdoors. You will want something that protects your baby's feet but still allows for some flexibility. For parents contemplating purchasing their baby's first shoes, here are some suggestions for things to consider:

* Make sure you get the proper fit. Shoes that are too tight or too loose could be painful or cause blisters and may even hamper walking. Have your pediatrician measure your child's feet during the regular check-ups. This will provide you with an accurate measurement.

* Avoid stiff, high-top leather shoes: there is no evidence that they help babies walk. Instead, look for something soft and flexible that allows your baby to use the movement of his feet to maintain balance and to walk. They should be made from canvas or some other breathable material and have flat, flexible, non-slip soles.

* Safe closures. Make sure that your baby's shoes fasten well. Double-knot laces so that they are less likely to come undone and make sure buckle straps are secure without being too tight.

* Get the shoe that is most comfortable for your child, even if it is not the same size that the measurement device indicates. Allow about one-half inch of space at the end of the longest toe to the end of the shoe. The toes should be able to wiggle freely, and the heel should not slip with normal walking. Inspect the shoe fit every couple of weeks to insure the continuing comfort of your child's feet.

Tricia O'Connell, special needs teacher and co-founder of Pip Squeakers
New Jersey

Put lightweight socks on your 2- to 3-week-old before the "stretchy" to help keep baby's legs in the "stretchy's" legs. This helps avoid the frantic baby who is entangled in his/her clothes.

Karen, doula and mother of Ross and Ian
Connecticut

Put a nightgown (the type that does not have any strings or snaps) on the baby at night. When you get up in the middle of the night, you want to make it quick for everyone; and if you have something with buttons or snaps, it takes longer when changing the diaper.

Georgeanne, labor and postpartum doula and mother of
four and grandmother of four
Maryland

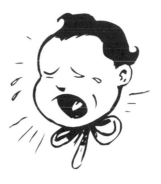

Crying

Crying is an infant's only form of communication. Infants are instinctively trying to express their needs: embrace it, respond to it, and you will create a happy being!

Alexis H, L&D nurse and mother of Caleb, 5 months
Illinois

If you have a colicky baby, it may help to swaddle the baby securely in a soft receiving blanket, rock baby, and whisper softly to him/her. Although baby may resist this initially, gradually this helps baby to calm down. As baby grows older, the whispering technique can be helpful to provide reassurance and a sense of calmness to your child during temper outbursts, clinging at times of separation, and many other stressful times.

Elizabeth B. Cusack, MA, NCSP, NJ, and nationally certified school psychologist, mother of Sean (and his wife Carrie), Maureen (and her husband Davin), and grandmother-to-be
New Jersey

Babies often cry because they need reassurance and to know where you are. Responding to babies' cries let them know they are important and that you are there for them. Newborns thrive on touch and being held. Babies who are held a lot cry less frequently.

Margot, RN, LCCE, CBE, and mother of
Mike, age 36, Stephanie, age 34, Jenny, age 32, and grandmother of five
Kansas

You can't spoil a baby. They learn to be loved by being held and snuggled and kissed and sung to. If you respond to your child's first cry, he/she knows you will be there whenever he/she needs you. It is the beginning of a trusting relationship.

**Elizabeth, part-time seamstress and full-time mother of
Erin, age 13, Kelly, age 10, Drew, age 7, and Caitlin, age 5
Massachusetts**

After my third colicky baby, I was thrilled to discover Dr. Harvey Karp's *The Happiest Baby on the Block*. For me, his tips provided the solutions I needed to soothe my fussy baby. I only wish I knew them 12 years earlier when my first was born!

**Debbie Glasser, licensed clinical psychologist, founder of www.newsforparents.org,
and mother of Emily, age 12, Ben, age 8, and Sam, age 2
Florida**

Crying is how babies talk to you. The best way to make it stop is to listen.

**Heather, mother of Ryleigh, age 4
Maryland**

An infant has one job in those first four months of life. Parents have one job in the first four months, too. The infant's job is to adjust to all the workings of a new body. At times it's very scary and frustrating to have a body, and I JUST NEED TO CRY. Crying is how babies let off steam. The parent's job is to respond to EVERY need a child has during the first four months. You CAN'T spoil an infant by responding to his/her EVERY need. Responding to EVERY need tells the child's psyche that the world is a safe place and can be trusted. EVERYTHING about emotions, bonding, and trust starts with those experiences. Don't let this information make you feel pressured. Follow your heart. Your heart is very attuned to your infant's needs – trust it. That trust is the beginning of parental intuition. You can hold a child as often as is needed during that time with no fear of spoiling. Any corrections you need to make to the constant holding or sleeping issues can be made after four months. You can get sleep and allow your child to cry if you need to. Dr. Karp's book *The Crying Baby* will help you with those issues. Dr. T. Berry Brazelton is the best authority to read about infancy and early childhood. Enjoy the formation of your new family.

**Sharon Silver, founder and director of The Center for Conscious Parenting,
www.cfcp.info, and mother of two glorious young adults
Oregon**

If your baby won't calm down, undress her and take your shirt off. Cuddle her against your chest, providing as much skin-to-skin contact as possible. If it's cold, use a blanket to cover you both, but don't break contact. This did wonders for my daughter when she was small.

Gessika, mother of Samantha, age 4
Maryland

Our first baby had colic. What a nightmare! My brother-in-law, Larry, told us this little tip he used with his five kids. Turn on the bathroom fan or stove vent fan and hold your baby nearby. The white noise of the fans was like magic. It was the best new parent advice I received.

Andrea, mother of Zachary, age 4, and Joshua, age 3
Texas

Sometimes a crying baby is just a little overwhelmed by everything and needs to cry to shut out the outside world for a little while. Shushing really works to quiet a crying baby because it helps the child cover any outside distractions that may be bothering him/her. Any other white noise will work, too. The dryer or vacuum were favorites of my daughter.

Heidi, courtesy of The Center for Conscious Parenting, www.cfcp.info,
"run-outside-of-the-house" mom and mother of Heather, age 20 months
Oregon

If you have fed and burped your baby and checked his/her diaper, don't worry about his/her crying! Take a shower or a short walk outside to recharge. It'll do wonders on your nerves.

Aggie, teacher and mother of Alexandra, age 2½, and Cassandra, 6 months
California

Always remember that you can't possibly spoil a baby. So many times we are told not to pick our children up when they are crying because they need to learn to be independent. Enjoy the cuddles! Cuddle them as much as you can and enjoy every second. Remember, one day, when they are 12 or 13, they will probably not even want to admit that they are even related to you.

Laila, work-at-home business consultant and mother of
Maria, age 2, and Matthew, age 4 months
British Columbia, Canada

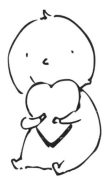

—Bonding with Baby—

Your baby spends months listening to your heartbeat and voice. The first few weeks after birth, your baby will prefer to be close to your skin listening to what he/she knows about you best…your heartbeat. Your baby listened to it beat fast and slow, and knew more about your heart than your face. But your baby is willing to learn the rest all from his/her place of comfort, snuggled at your chest.

Amanda, stay-at-home mother of Samantha Alexis, age 11 months
Ohio

I think the best advice I got came from interviewing so many families who made everyday rituals a priority. Little things like bedtime rituals have made me much closer to my son. Even the silly ritual we do in the morning when he gets his vitamin makes life more fun: I get him Flintstone vitamins; and every single day I'll say what character the vitamin is shaped like, and Max will insist that "It's Dino" (a dinosaur), no matter what. We both insist and just get silly about it.

Meg Cox, author of *The Book of New Family Traditions* and mother of Max, age 9
New Jersey

Start massaging your baby as soon as he's born. It relaxes him, he'll sleep better, and it's great for overall development.

Geraldine Hickey, RN, owner of Two-Fit, www.two-fit.com
New Jersey

You never know who your children will become, so love them with an open mind and open heart and without expectations. It is the most fun to just enjoy them for the unique, special person that they are becoming. Above all else, take good care of yourself and have as much fun with them as you can!

Deborah, psychologist and mother of Alex, age 30, and Sally, age 28
California

When Mom holds the baby, baby gets a somatosensory bath (Dr. Bruce Perry) which means baby can smell you, feel you, taste you, hear you, and gaze into your eyes. Babies are not high tech. Their needs are pretty basic: touch, eye contact, warm milk (preferably breast milk, if that works for you), the sound of your voice, rocking, and dry diapers.

Margot, RN, LCCE, CBE, and mother of
Mike, age 36, Stephanie, age 34, Jenny, age 32, and grandmother of five
Kansas

Don't forget infant massage! Touch is key to your infant's development, from gas and colic relief to communicating your love and comfort.

Aimee, certified pre/postnatal and infant massage therapist
Illinois

I massage my girls every night using Johnson and Johnson bedtime lotion. I start from the back of their necks all the way to their toes. I swear they sleep like little angels.

Cathy, nurse and mother of Niki, age 3, Marina, age 1, and Baby # 3 due in April
New Jersey

The best advice is to follow your instincts! It's natural for a mother to want to be around her baby all the time; to pick up her baby as soon as he/she cries, because everyone wants a cuddle when they cry; to breastfeed and to sleep together. Be as possessive of your baby as you want to be: completely bond with your baby; do all in your power to breastfeed, which is the first thing that you and baby learn to do together (you wouldn't become a mechanic without first learning to fix a car); sleep together, which cements the mother-child bond. And lastly, pick up your baby every time he/she cries, because everyone cries for a reason. (This gives the baby the knowledge that all needs will be met.)

Tracy, mother of Kole, age 14, Jessica, age 3, and Taylor, age 1
Mt Roskill, Auckland, New Zealand

Make up a special song with your child's name and sing it to him/her everyday. It is amazing how this will calm and reassure your child. My boys still like me to sing "their" song every night.

Heidi, portfolio manager and mother of Christian, age 9, and Nathan, age 6
Nevada

Get in the tub with your baby. It's easier to hold him, and you get two clean, happy people for the price of one!

Liesl, professor of chemistry and mother of Liam, age 8 months
New Jersey

Baby massage is great for them to relax and for digestion/gas and just fun Mommy-and-baby time. With fingers together, place your pinky side just above their bellybutton (thumb up towards you) and stroke gently down right hand then left (one after the other). Another is to lay your hands, palms down, on the tummy and just use a three fingers to make a heart shape up and around to their chest and V down to their belly button. Then massaging too their arms and legs.

Courtesy of the moms of Blackberry Creek Community Church in Aurora, IL

You can never give a child too much love. Cuddles, kisses, and touches are very important to their development. Don't be afraid to cuddle, hug, love, rock, and hold your baby. You cannot spoil them this way. Remember to relax and ENJOY your baby. You will never have this moment again, whatever it is, because tomorrow your baby will be a day older; and that is one less day you have together. Sit back, take all the cuddles you can get, and let your baby bring you all the joy!!

Angela, stay-at-home mother of
Brittany, age 11, Gabrielle, age 10, Kassandra, age 7, Isabela, age 5, and Danijela 1
Virginia

This takes time, honestly. Make it a point to read a short nursery rhyme at each feeding as you finish, even if baby is asleep. I now take my 6-month-old into the shower with me. We tend to sit on the shower floor and play with the falling "rain." I get to have some fun playtime with her while I grab a shower. But the best part is that I am holding her close to me, just the two of us, for those few minutes.

Christine, full-time diva and mother of Julia, age 2½, and Olivia, age 6 months
New Jersey

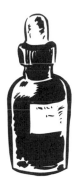

$\int$ick $\int$aby

The absolute best cure for diarrhea is chamomile tea. Simply brew as you would with a tea bag, let cool, and mix ¾ tea with ¼ juice or Gatorade.

**Sheryl Fernandez, owner of Bellies and Bubbles Maternity
and mother of Dalton, age 16 months
Pennsylvania**

My son had chronic diarrhea later in his first year. After the first bout, I thought I was free, but oh no. To calm the stomach but still give him nutrition, I fed him scrambled eggs (whites only), clear chicken broth, boiled chicken, and lots of water (to clean out the system and prevent diaper rash). NO MILK, milk products, or regular formula was given. Consult a physician if diarrhea lasts more than a couple of days. (My son's lasted four months; I also discovered the value of old plastic pants.) It could be something more serious. Thankfully, mine was just teething.

**Deedy, mother of David
Oklahoma**

If your newborn has a low grade fever, and you hate the idea of putting cold packs on him, peel a head of cold lettuce and stuff his clothes. The fever will usually be gone by the time the lettuce is wilted!

**LeeAlice, mother of Colt Ashton and Cannon Avery, age 3
Texas**

When baby is sick, a BATH to the rescue! The bath water should be about your baby's temperature (if he/she has a fever), and it will equalize baby's circulation. Your baby will feel better, take a nice nap, and recover quickly. I would do this three or four times a day when my children got sick. Also, giving baby a quick cold dash rub with a soppy wash cloth will close the pores and prevent chilling. Your baby may resist, but in the end, he/she will feel much better because he/she will not get cold. This also has the ability to strengthen the immune system.

Phoebe, RN, LCCE, mother of Marie, age 37, Craig, age 34, Michelle, age 33, and Marsha, age 32, and grandmother of Gabriella, age 13, Matthias, age 10, Erik, age 7, James, age 7, Ethan, age 5, Alek, age 4, Caleb, age 18 months, Andrew, age 17 months, and Zachary, age 13 months
Tennessee

When your doctor tells you how much medication to give, write it on the bottle with the date. That way, everyone knows what dose to give without looking for a paper. I have also highlighted a toddler dose with a highlighter pen. This also works well if you are giving the medicine to a sitter to administer. Remember that most doses are given related to the child's weight, so put the weight on the medicine bottle.

Dolores, R.N., Lamaze (LCCE), doula, and mother of Jonathon and Megan
New York

Please research vaccines. Our children need our wisdom and protection. If you can avoid it, do not vaccinate your child until after six months of age.

Michelle, registered nurse and mother of
Hannah, age 8, Saul, age 6, Jon, age 3, and Susan, age 4 months
Massachusetts

Before you just "go along" with having your children vaccinated, there are many things you should be aware of. Health issues possibly linked to vaccination include ADHD, asthma, autism, and now cancer in later years. Why isn't much more published about this? Just curious to see if there is any truth in the information I was given against vaccination.

Linda, godmother
Pennsylvania

Make sure you have an easy-to-read and understand first aid book handy with the pages on choking, fevers, burns, etc., tabbed with post-its so you can easily find the pages in an emergency situation.

Sherry Bonelli, owner www.mommysthinkin.com, and mother of Connor, age 6, and twins Sidney and Kiley, age 2
Illinois

After Taylor's fourth time having been on antibiotics, at age 5 he started complaining about his knees hurting. By that night after returning home from my multiples meeting, my husband asked if I had noticed Taylor's rash. I went in and noticed he had a rash and his joints were swollen. After a trip to the emergency room, we discovered it takes time for an allergy to form in the body. So from one day to the next he could no longer take penicillin. He identical brother, Tyler, is at a higher risk of forming an allergy as well; but, luckily, he hasn't as of yet.

Janet, homemaker and mother of identical twins Tyler and Taylor, age 8
Georgia

I made a homemade first aid kit stocked with gauze, tape, scissors, Band-aids, alcohol wipes, Neosporin, antibacterial gel, calamine lotion, anti-itch cream, a mini bottle of peroxide, hydrocortisone cream (1%), thermometer, tweezers, aloe vera gel, list of emergency numbers, first aid instructions for any injury that a child may sustain, list of dosing recommendations for age and weight, infants' Tylenol and Motrin, and instant cold packs. I packed all of this in an old baby wipes container (they're absolutely FABULOUS for storage and organizing). I also made a travel first aid kit with just the essentials and used a travel wipes container which fits easily in the glove box of the car.

Lori, former preschool teacher, now stay-at-home mother of Jeffrey, age 6 months
Illinois

Take common sense precautions to prevent accidents and the onset of illnesses.
Beverly, teacher and mother of three sons
Tennessee

Take a stand when it comes to your child's health. I am the mother of four, including twin daughters. My greatest challenge was the birth of my youngest son, who was obviously sick at birth. He was a couple of weeks early and jaundice in color. After several days in an isolet and on monitors, the doctor felt that his breathing had stabilized and sent him home. The second night at home, he wouldn't nurse. You could tell he was struggling to breathe. I waited for sunrise and called my doctor. They gave him an 11 am appointment. But a short time later he turned purple in my arms, and I called the office and said I was bringing him NOW! I remember, my oldest, age 5, couldn't find his shoes so I took him and the twins (who were three) to the neighbors in his slippers in the snow and drove the baby to the doctor's office. My baby quit breathing again in the doctor's office, and they took us by ambulance to Children's Hospital. Scott was 2 weeks old. He was hooked up to all kinds of tubes and monitors, given an antibiotic, and was kept for 28 days. We were all traumatized, but thankfully he responded and again came home. The antibiotic had killed off all the natural bacteria in his mouth, and for three months we administered more medicine for thrush. When I finally had enough, I refused to get another prescription! A doctor who had worked in the Peace Corp asked if I could get the baby to take yogurt. I expressed my breast milk and added the yogurt. It took a little prodding but he drank it and got well! A natural remedy for the medicine! Sometimes you need to take a stand! I am so gratefully that Scott is alive and healthy today!

**Madonna, mental health therapist and mother of
Sean, twins Penny and Nikki, and Scott
Ohio**

Visitors rule: wash your hands and no kissing! It's probably one of the hardest things to ask of your family members, but it will save you the ordeal of a sick baby. I knew to ask everyone to wash his or her hands. I'd heard it from veteran moms and the pediatrician. My son was born in December, smack in the middle of flu season. I felt very proud of myself for monitoring everyone's hand-washing until I found my son showered with wet kisses. Ugh! Now what? I changed the rules to include the "no kissing" clause.

**Michele, freelance writer and mother
Colorado**

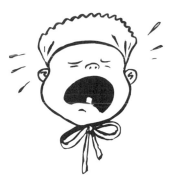

Teething

I have found that running a washcloth under very warm water, wringing it out, and letting my daughter chew on it is better for her gums than using something cold. The warmth of the washcloth seems to soften her gums rather than make them harder by using something cold. I also used this technique with my son when he was teething as a baby. It really helped!

Ramanda, stay-at-home mother of Wesson, age 4½, and Gracie, age 8 months
Arkansas

When my baby was teething, she loved a frozen washcloth. I would wet it and then shape it into a ring so it was easy for her little hands to hold. Once she started getting more teeth around 6 months, she liked small chipped ice. She would just hold it in her mouth and let it melt or chew on it. Nursing her frequently helped ease her pain and comfort her: the breast pressed to her gums felt good. This was a big help at night. She would just fall asleep next to me in bed while nursing and could have access to me whenever she wanted. Also, a product called Angel Brush from UBB helped us during this time. It's a little tooth brush for teething and brushing baby's first teeth. My baby would chew on this for an hour at a time. It's shaped in a small curve that fits perfectly in the side of her mouth.

Lisa, stay-at-home mother of Abby, age 10 months
South Carolina

Three tips...

1. Chill your baby's pacifier in the fridge to soothe sore gums.

2. Chilled water or milk in a bottle can also be soothing/numbing for a sore mouth.

3. Don't wait until the pain is really bad to give pain relief. Keep up a continuous dose of a pain reliever, such as Tylenol, to help head off the pain before it begins.

Susanna Bartee, founder and editor of www.militarymama.net, and full-time mother of Abigail, age 11, Hannah, age 8, Hank, age 6, and Lucy, age 1
Germany

The best teether I've found is The First Years Massaging Action Teether. After trying everything else, this was the only thing that provided some relief to my teething infant. I kept it in the fridge so it would be chilled, too.

Rebecca, insurance trainer and mother of Allye, age 13, and Addie, age 2
Texas

A wise pediatrician gave me this bit of advice 30 years ago, and it works! Diaper rash is not caused by acid. It happens because when a baby is teething, he/she drools out important enzymes that neutralize the alkali. Dilute grape juice with water and give this to baby once a day, especially during teething.

Karen, secretary and mother of Jeffrey, age 33, and Lori, age 30
Rhode Island

My baby really liked teething on frozen bagels. She just carried them around the house, and the mess was minimal.

Kristi, therapist and mother of Zoe, age 15 months
Texas

Saline drops! The nerves from a person's top teeth run along the nasal passages. This can be painful, especially when teething. Give baby a mist of baby nasal saline spray, especially before bed. It will help alleviate any pressure and let everyone get a better rest without the use of additional drugs.

Margaret, homemaker and mother of Braden, age 4
Texas

Fill a nipple with water, put the stopper on, and freeze it to make a nipple pop teether! (Avent bottles work especially well.)

Stacey, anthropologist and mother of Satchel, age 2, and Jiro, age 5 months
Tennessee

Freeze fruits to put in a baby-safe net feeder. It soothes their gums and tastes yummy. Also try freezing one end of a washcloth, keeping the other end unfrozen for their hands. My son loved these tricks.

Melodie, stay-at-home mother of Cameron Drew, age 4
Florida

Babies are not born with the bacteria that cause tooth decay and gum infections. Bacteria are transmitted through saliva. Kissing, cups, utensils, and unwashed hands are carriers of millions of germs. When sampling baby's food, never put utensils into your mouth then into baby's. Always use a clean spoon, even if you have to put several in the diaper bag.

Sheila Wolf, registered dental hygienist, author of *Pregnancy and Oral Health: The Critical Connection Between Your Mouth and Your Baby*, and mother of Alan, age 31

A mother can greatly influence a child's dental habits by cleaning baby's teeth as soon as they appear in the mouth. Usually between 5 and 8 months, the lower front teeth (incisors) will begin to push through the gums – a bit earlier for girls than boys. Using a soft, wet facecloth, a piece of sterile gauze, or a very soft toothbrush (NOT an old one of yours), you can clean the soft plaque off baby's newly erupting teeth. Since teething sometimes makes baby very irritable, something cool and wet is often helpful to soothe those tender gums. My favorite recipe that offers both comfort and nutrition is homemade popsicles. Take one 6-ounce can of orange juice concentrate, mix with an 8-ounce container of plain yogurt, and freeze until solid. Yummy!

Sheila Wolf, registered dental hygienist, author of *Pregnancy and Oral Health: The Critical Connection Between Your Mouth and Your Baby* and mother of Alan, age 31

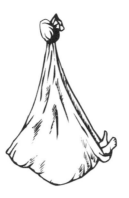

Baby Slings

Wear your baby!

Morgan, mother of Kieran, age 17 months
New York

Hold your baby as much as possible, especially during the first six months. Invest in a quality baby carrier. Your child will feel more secure, meet this need earlier, and be able to assert his independence at the appropriate age. You will never regret the time you spend together with your baby.

Sherry, registered nurse and mother of Mitchell, age 4, and Mia, age 2
Indiana

Slings are more than carrying devices. They can be a hammock that holds your baby at breast level for nursing (great for when you nurse while standing or sitting in a straight-back chair or on a bench at the park), helps you nurse discreetly, and keeps your baby warm (fleece ones especially). Slings can also offer protection from the sun (Solarveil) and can double as a blanket for lying on the grass or swaddling during a nap. There are many different varieties…I encourage internet shopping for the best selection.

Karen Laing, lactation consultant, owner of Birthways Doula Services in Chicago, and mother of Birkleigh, age 9 months
Illinois

With a very wakeful baby I walked around holding him in a sling and in a baby hammock so I could get things done as he didn't like being away from me. It also was a comfort when he was having trouble sleeping through the night to know that it's a stage, and it won't last forever.

Jacinda, domestic goddess and mother of
Hamish, age 4, and George, age 18 months
New Zealand

Use a sling to carry baby. Chances are you're going to carry your baby most of the time anyway, especially if there are other children at home. This way you can still have your hands somewhat free.

Jessica, mother of Steven, age 6, Olivia, age 5, and George, age 2
New Jersey

Wear your baby in a sling or wrap! Babies fuss less when carried and love being physically close to your body. You can get things done around the house while your baby naps. I use a Moby wrap with Mya, and she loves it. It's also great exercise carrying a baby, which helps shed the pregnancy pounds.

Jayati, mother of Mya, age 8 months
Ontario, Canada

We found that the challenges of caring for a newborn (and beyond) were made so much easier by breastfeeding, co-sleeping, and using a sling. The result for us was that our daughter rarely cried.

Sherri, mother of Emma, age 3½
New York

Invest in a comfortable, good quality baby sling. They're absolutely essential for a "high needs" baby! You'll be able to give your baby the closeness and attention your baby deserves while leaving your hands free to clean, care for other children, shop for groceries, or just go for a walk. They're also great for discreet nursing. Mine was a lifesaver, and my daughter loved it! She still asks for "slinging" at age 2, and I'm happy to oblige.

Shawna, mother of Kaylee, age 2
Michigan

My baby loved the sling. Most of the time it put her right to sleep and kept her happy for hours. I could get so much done, and Daddy loved to wear her, too! It also makes nursing baby very easy and helps conceal nursing. You just use the tail of the sling to cover baby and your exposed breast. Now that she is older, I use a baby carrier. The one I use and love is an Asian baby carrier. This type of carrier keeps her facing my chest and the straps cross in the back for back support. Again, my baby loves to be close to me, and I love being hands free and stroller free. It's a godsend for places like Disney: you don't have to park a stroller or put her to sleep – she just snuggles up to you, and she's out! It also keeps her happy and warm in cold weather.

Lisa, stay-at-home mother of Abby, age 10 months
South Carolina

Get a sling or front pack and wear your baby! It makes everyone's life easier.

Jesse, teacher
Oregon

Wearing your baby in a sling is a great way to keep your baby close, soothe a colicky baby, nurse and shop at the same time, and feel your baby's warmth with your hands free.

Terese, infant sign instructor and mother of
a girl, age 4½, and a boy, age 2
Alberta, Canada

Hold your baby as much as possible, and invest in a great sling like an Asian baby carrier or pouch. Don't become a "baby car seat carrier." Car seats are for cars only, not for carrying your baby – your arms are for that!

Heather, registered nurse
South Carolina

Wait until just AFTER the baby is born to be fitted for a sling (or nursing bra). Find out in advance who specializes in slings and will help with fitting you and your baby once your baby is born. Slings differ for height and comfort for each person and baby. My advice: skip the big stroller and wear your baby as much as possible!

Margaret, homemaker and mother of Braden, age 4
Texas

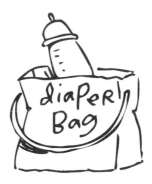

Packing a Baby Bag

I always keep a diaper bag fully stocked and ready to go by the door, so the only thing I have to do is grab a sippy cup or bottle. All snacks are in baggies inside in a master zipper lock bag so they keep. Getting the kids together is hard enough; rechecking the diaper bag is one less thing to have to deal with.

**Christine, full-time diva and mother of Julia, age 2½, and Olivia, age 6 months
New Jersey**

Always repack the bag (including zipper lock bags of snacks) as soon as you can after you get home. That way, it'll be ready to go the next time you are headed out the door. This is especially helpful if you are in a hurry and cannot stop to check what needs to be replaced. You'll also be doing it when you're not as stressed and can remember everything that needs to be replaced.

**Carole, owner of KidTime Charlotte (drop-in child care center) and mother of
Jake, age 5, and Connor, age 21 months
North Carolina**

Use a backpack instead of an over-the-shoulder diaper bag. That way you have both hands free for the baby, groceries, opening doors, etc.

**Heidi, courtesy of The Center for Conscious Parenting, www.cfcp.info,
"run-outside-of-the-house" mom and mother of Heather, age 20 months
Oregon**

I sprinkle some powder in a diaper wrapped in the changing cloth for trips — less bulk in the bag. Use plastic zipper bags for wipes and snacks instead of containers. They also eliminate bulk and are disposable.

**Tara, high school teacher and at-home-mother of Kiley, age 2
California**

Always keep a diaper bag packed and by the door with a couple of diapers, wipes, and a change of clothes! When I am about to go nuts and need out of the house, I am very thankful for that packed bag.

**Kiera, student and mother of Audrey, age 2
Oregon**

Always keep a supply of plastic zipper lock bags in your diaper bag. The gallon-size ones are the best, although I've been known to carry around a bunch of different sizes. I have used them countless times and continue to use them even though my kids are out of diapers! They are perfect for so many things: wet clothes, dirty diapers (It's amazing how many times we've been places where there are no garbage cans.), extra wipes, leftover food, dividing up a snack (Have you ever seen two children try to share one bag of goldfish crackers?), empty juice boxes and other trash, holding small toys (i.e., Polly Pockets and her multitude of tiny clothes and shoes), dry paper towels and tissues, etc. They are also helpful for slipping over your hands if you have to clean up something particularly messy. The gallon-size bags are also fantastic for packing kids' clothes for traveling. Just place one whole outfit into each bag (i.e., shirt, pants, underwear, socks, hair accessories) and then when it's time to get dressed, there's no hunting around the suitcase for the wayward socks or headbands. When the outfits are packed this way, they also lay flat, which gives you more packing room. The bags can even be labeled with the child's name and/or the day or occasion for which the outfit was packed. Whenever I give a baby shower gift, I always include a box of zipper lock bags. In my opinion, they are indispensable.

**Rachel, mother of Sarah, age 5, and Ben, age 4
Massachusetts**

Keep two diaper bags packed and ready at all times. Leave one by the front door.

**Dolores, R.N., Lamaze (LCCE), doula, and mother of Jonathon and Megan
New York**

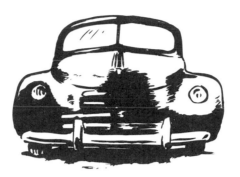

Getting Out

Keep an extra diaper bag in your car with diapers, wipes, and a change of clothes. That way, you can get out of the house fast when you need to. Remember to restock the bag after it has been used.

**Jennifer, Lakeland Parents of Multiples and mother of
Becki, age 14, Sarah, age 12, and Andrew and Elizabeth, age 6**

When at the grocery store, park right next to the cart corral. That way, you don't have to carry the baby all the way inside to get a cart; and when you finish shopping, you can feel safe putting the car seat in the car while you empty the groceries and put the cart back.

**Tracy, director of Christian education and mother of
Hannah, age 2, and Christian, age 4 months
Pennsylvania**

Throw a sheet on the floor of your car when traveling with infants or toddlers to help protect your car from those inevitable messes. When you get home, simply take out the sheet and shake it out and throw it in the washing machine.

**Kim Danger, owner www.mommysavers.com, and mother of
Sydney, age 5, and Nicholas, age 1
Minnesota**

If it's any other season than winter, after your baby reaches 4 to 6 weeks old, strap him/her into your carrier (on your body – I liked the Bay Bjorn) and go for a walk. It's a great way to have peaceful time with your new baby, give yourself an exercise treat, and enjoy the beautiful weather. Your baby will love to snuggle in close to you, hear your heartbeat, and enjoy to gentle motion of walking.

Melinda, full-time mother of Georgia, age 5, and Charley, age 16 months
Maryland

Don't get dressed to go anywhere until AFTER you've fed, burped, and changed baby. I'm sure you're carrying an extra outfit or two for baby, but why don't you pack one for yourself to keep in the car? I was sitting in the middle of a children's museum when my baby, who I was trying to nurse discreetly, had a blowout poop and leaked through his diaper, outfit, and right onto me!

Elisabeth K. Corcoran, author of *Calm in my Chaos: Encouragement for a Mom's Weary Soul* (Kregel Publications, www.kregel.com), and mother of Sarah, age 7½, and Jack, age 6
Illinois

Instead of carrying lots of necessities in the diaper bag and adding to the weight, have a couple of bags in your trunk — one filled with toys only taken to parks or restaurants and the other with backup diapers, first aid kits, change of clothes, etc.

Angela, homemaker and mother of Dylan, age 10, and Nicholas, age 1½
California

Our daughter had a very hard time in the car until a friend recommended nursing her in her car seat…what a difference it made. It takes a little gymnastic maneuver, but it's worth it!

Sherri, mother of Emma, age 3½
New York

Have a box of toys in the front seat for times when your baby drops his/hers. It will keep him/her busy and happy while traveling!

Kelly, StrollerFit specialist and mother of Isabella, age 1
Texas

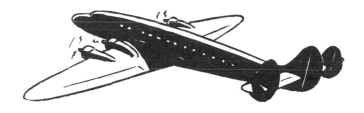

— Traveling with Baby —

Baby powder is magical when on the beach with children. If you sprinkle some on your hand and rub your child's body with it where the sand is, the sand easily wipes away. This is by far the BEST tip I have ever received.

Christie, mother of Jackson, age 4, and Mackenzie, age 5 months
New Jersey

While doing research on how best to travel with a baby, I found this great company called Baby's Away that rents baby gear. They delivered the crib right to our destination and picked it up when we were finished.

It was by far the easiest way to have the comforts of home while traveling. Besides cribs, you can rent strollers, car seats, etc. I would recommend the company to anyone with small kids who like to travel.

Mary, mother of Julia, age 9, and Mitchell, 8 months
Ohio

Babies under the age of two fly free on most airlines. However, if you do decide to purchase a seat for your child, don't forget to enroll him or her in a frequent flier program. Even infants can start accumulating frequent flier miles to use towards free airline tickets.

Kim Danger, owner www.mommysavers.com, and mother of
Sydney, age 5, and Nicholas, age 1
Minnesota

When traveling with baby, always have a small "medical emergency kit" that includes a thermometer, notepad and pen, Infant's or Children's Tylenol or Motrin with dose chart, and your child's weight in pounds and kilograms. When flying, load your carry-on bag with the following: the number of diapers you think you'll need times two, wipes, zipper lock bags, changing pad, breast pads, a small bottle of baby wash and a washcloth, and appropriate food for you and baby. In the car or in your luggage, it's helpful to always have zipper lock bags, at least 15 diapers, baby wash and wipes, and a change of clothes for you and baby. And remember — don't immunize your child the week before you are traveling.

Brooke A. Schumacher, M.D., and mother of a daughter, age 3, and twin sons, age 1½
Dhahran, Saudi Arabia

Pack a pair of pajamas, no matter what age your child is; then you can stay at friends' house that little bit longer and dress your child before leaving. It means no more waking your child up to get ready for bed.

Elizabeth, nursery nurse and mother of Rowan (as in tree), age 13 weeks

Buy a tiny paddling pool from a cheap shop and a plastic tea set or little containers. While you lie back and sunbathe, your little one (as long as he/she can sit up) will play safely for hours beside you while you drape one hand in the water to check on him/her!

Angela, headhunter and mother of Jazmin, age 12, and Amber, age 9
Garden Suburb, United Kingdom

We do a lot of traveling on weekends to visit family. To help pass the time we keep our daughter's favorite CD in the car and a small backpack with toys. She only sees these toys when in the car, so when she opens the bag, it is like they are brand new to her. I think it is also comforting. She knows that when she gets in the car she can hear "Silly Songs with Larry," read some books, and play with familiar toys.

Kristine, pampered chef consultant and mother of Isabel, age 2
Pennsylvania

Be sure to pack an extra T-shirt for yourself on the airplane! I have found myself in situations where I have the extra outfit for baby in case of an accident but nothing for myself.

Annie, designer and mother of Emma, age 5½, and Sophie, age 3
California

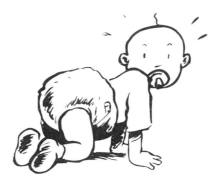

Development

Babies need flat, firm surfaces and uncluttered space to stretch and grow and develop at their own pace. Give your baby plenty of time on the floor both on the back and on the tummy. Lying on the tummy helps strengthen neck and back muscles. It gives babies a chance to learn to hold their own weight through their arms, which will become strong enough for crawling later. It also adds a new perspective to the rooms that they are in. Some babies do not like being on their tummy and will show their dislike by crying or becoming frustrated. If your baby is like this, a few suggestions are:

· get down on the floor with him/her for a while
· catch his/her interest with a toy and place both baby and toy down together
· roll up a towel or pillow and prop baby up under his/her shoulders with his/her elbows in front of it

From mothers of children who are volunteers of the Bonnie Babes Foundation Victoria, Australia

Refrain from revealing your concerns over any developmental delays your child may be experiencing to playgroup friends. Moms are extremely competitive, and, unfortunately, some moms use the information as a comparison that leaves your child stigmatized and labeled. Instead, consult only with close friends and family, your pediatrician, or read books to alleviate your concerns. And remember, your child will be all caught up by kindergarten anyway.

Karen, homemaker and mother of Dylan, age 2, and Shelby, age 4 months

During foot development, it is important for bones, muscles, blood vessels, and nerves to have room to grow without restriction. As the beginning walker stands up and takes his first tentative steps, the muscles of his feet grip the floor, and the toes separate to help the child have better balance and control. If his feet are confined within a rigid shoe, the toes cannot operate in this way nor can the muscles of the foot and ankle develop the strength necessary to hold him upright. Soft-soled baby shoes allow the beginning walker to grip the floor, developing strong ankles and flexible foot bones. This creates a solid foundation for bone and muscle formation in the rest of the body, especially the spinal column. A level pelvis and straight spine depend upon healthy feet throughout our entire lives, beginning in infancy.

Lisa C. Moore, Doctor of Chiropractic
California

Don't read too many books on child rearing. Many times you will find that the advice givers contradict each other. And too much information can make you feel inadequate and second guess yourself. Take one day at a time and let your children be who they are. Don't worry about stopping the pacifier or the bottle, sleeping in your bed, or being potty trained by age 2½. (Both of my daughters are none the worse for following THEIR schedules on all four of those – which were not "by the book"!) Drop the neurosis. Your child will not suffer if he/she does not follow the so-called "experts" timeline. Your child will not do it forever; we all grow up. Remember, every child is different and will follow his/her own schedule whether you like it or not. Revel in your child's unique individuality. Welcome to the most rewarding job you will ever have.

Cindy, mother of Caeley, age 6, and Cameron, age 4
California

Certain sounds are expected to be developed at certain ages.
Ages 2½ to 3 years — m, p, w, t
Ages 3 to 3½ years — b, d
Ages 3½ to 4 years — k, g, f
Ages 4 to 4½ years — s, sh, j, ch, z
Ages 4½ to 5 years — v, l
Ages 5 to 7 years — r, th blends

Elaine Emily Dreyfuss, speech pathologist and mother of Emil, age 7
New Jersey

So, you think your child may not be developing appropriately? Follow your maternal instinct. Don't be embarrassed. Don't deny a potential problem. If you sense a problem, have your child evaluated by a neurologist, developmental pediatrician, or at the very least, your local Early Intervention (or other county or state) Agency. What is the harm in doing so? If you panicked unnecessarily, no harm done. The evaluations are painless, non-intrusive, and if performed by the appropriate Early Intervention or other governmental agency, they are free. Our children think they are merely playing during these evaluations! If you are right, however, and your child does have developmental concerns, research clearly shows that the earlier one intervenes, the greater chance of success in addressing the concerns. And remember, your child may or may not "qualify" for free special educational services under state and federal law. That is a different issue than whether or not your child has needs that require intervention by a therapist of some nature.

You are your child's best advocate. Trust your instinct. Get informed about your child's issues. Look for support in your friends, family, and local organizations and support groups, easily located on the internet or through your state Department of Education. If you have been blessed with a child that may have some unique or challenging needs beyond the "typical" youngster, it is probably because God knew you would rise to the challenge and take care of your little one! I say this as a mom similarly blessed by my daughter, who with the help of intensive therapy since she was 18 months old, just started kindergarten in a classroom containing typical children! And remember, record your child's strengths as well as her weaknesses through her development. Video her monthly and keep a journal. This will not only provide a record for experts who evaluate your child in the future but also allows you to look back and see how much progress your child has really made.

Patricia, housewife, attorney, and mother of
Kaitlin, age 5, and Ashley, age 3½
New York

Difficult though it may be, try very hard to resist the temptation to compare your baby to other babies his/her age or to the charts in baby books that tell you when your baby "should" roll over, crawl, etc. Every baby is an individual and develops at his or her own speed. Just try to enjoy watching your baby grow and change without worrying about when baby will do the next big thing. Baby will do it when ready and not a second before.

Julia, stay-at-home mother of Lysander, age 7 months
New Jersey

Important pediatric studies conclude that children should walk barefoot in order to allow their feet to develop naturally. When weather and conditions make barefoot walking impractical, soft-soled shoes are the next best choice as they allow your child's feet to flex naturally while your child is learning to walk or crawl. Leading podiatrists agree that well-fastened soft-soled shoes are better for your baby when taking those first important steps and for some months afterwards. When choosing a size for your little one, make sure there is at least a quarter-inch room to grow.

Bettina Rasmussen and Amy Browne, co-owners of PlatyPaws Soft Soles Baby Shoes
and mothers of Dylan, age 3 (Bettina), and Owen, age 3,
and Isabella, age 9 months (Amy)
California

With my first born, Bella, my husband and I couldn't wait for her to reach each milestone. It was like we counted down the days until the next milestone arrived. As the first year came and went we realized how quickly it flew by. With our second child, Gavin, my husband and I agreed that we wouldn't pay attention to when he should be reaching milestones. We would enjoy each and every day and not worry about what and if he'll reach the next milestone. When my son arrived two months early, we knew that we definitely wanted to live each day to the fullest and not focus on when he'll sit up, eat solids, or crawl. We knew that being a very premature baby he could be very behind. Much to our dismay our son is reaching his milestones just the way he's supposed to. I would say to my husband, "Gosh, that came quick," but then I knew, because we weren't putting so much energy into when he'll do certain things, that they just started to come up out of nowhere. I feel like we're not rushing the first year with him. My advice to you is to please not worry about when your friend's baby did this or that or what the books say. Just relax and enjoy each day and be mesmerized by the sparkle in your child's eye each time he/she discovers something new.

Jennifer, mother of Bella, age 2, and Gavin, age 9 months
Florida

Resist the temptation to compare your child's accomplishments, development, or behavior with others. There are plenty of ways to feel superior to the rest of the human race. Let the children stay innocent of that sin a little while longer.

Jennifer, accountant and mother of
Alex, age 9, Veronica, age 4, and Matthew, age 2
Minnesota

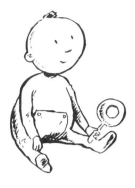

— Playing with Baby —

Take time everyday, even if it is just 15 minutes during bath time, to play with your baby. He/She won't want to play with you forever, so enjoy it while you can.

Beckie, mother of Alyssa, 10 months
Texas

Spend some time each day down on the floor with your infant, on a soft quilt or blanket, doing whatever he/she is doing.

Rev. Enid L. Ross, minister and hospital chaplain and mother of
Luke, age 21, Julia, age 17, and Celia, age 13
Texas

Never try to make a happy baby happier. When your baby, toddler, or child of any age is perfectly content doing what they're doing and what they're doing is safe and appropriate, don't go looking for something else to do instead. We are so conditioned to entertain our children that we often miss the value of letting them entertain themselves. We can lessen the stress on ourselves by letting them enjoy a chosen activity as long as it lasts.

Jennifer Elin Cole, author of *I Love You All the Time* and mother of
Mollie, age 6, Sophie, age 3, and Alan, age 3
Georgia

Take an empty 20-ounce or smaller plastic soda bottle, wash it and let it dry, then put rice in it. It makes a great rattle or teether, and you won't be upset when your baby loses it on a shopping trip.

Ruthann, stay-at-home mother of Mike, age 7, and Sarah, age 5
Maryland

I am always amazed at how content my son is to just watch me do things. We are always told that babies should be learning things and playing with educational toys that we forget that it is stimulating for them to just watch us. Having Jacob with me relaxes me because I know where he is, and it keeps him content and engaged.

Nicole, client services coordinator and mother of Jacob, age 8 months
New Jersey

These are fun things to have for baby playtime…

1. black and white activity gym or anything with dangling toys that baby can lie on the floor and look at

2. swing — perfect so that you and Dad can have a meal together, but don't let it become a sleep prop

3. touch and feel board books; board books with baby faces

4. bouncy seat with dangling toys — avoid using the vibrate motion as a routine soother or sleep prop

5. heartbeat animal — has a recording that sounds like the heartbeat in the womb — very soothing to baby; helpful when traveling because this was one more way to make a strange room feel familiar

6. long playing music — some baby equipment (mobiles, fake aquariums) have very short playtimes with the recordings. Check this out because 5 to 10 minutes is never long enough and you don't want to have to reset it.

7. CD player that attaches to the crib or one for the room

8. Symphony in Motion Mobile — twice as expensive as the Fisher Price one but so worth it. Our baby watched it for 20 to 25 minutes at a time from 8 weeks through 6 months. A lifesaver when you want to take a shower.

9. Mommy and Daddy are the best playthings!

The contributing moms of "The List," a growing list of
new mom tips passed from friend to friend
New Jersey, Maryland, and Delaware

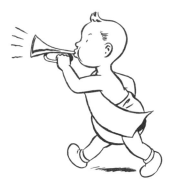

— Talking with Baby —

Your baby can recognize and is comforted by your voice from a very early age. By cooing, singing, and talking to your baby, it helps promote intellectual and language development. Opportunities for talking to your baby include bath time, nappy (diaper) change, shopping, drives in the car, and meal times, to name a few. If you talk in the "here and now," your baby will learn to associate words with objects or actions. You should speak slowly and clearly and focus on a single word of interest: "Look at the dog." "The dog is chasing the ball." "Look, the dog is running."

From mothers of children who are volunteers of the Bonnie Babes Foundation
Victoria, Australia

I once volunteered in a day care when I was very young. We were instructed to use only positive vocabulary on the property. I learned some very valuable lessons in how effective this way of speaking to children and other adults really is. It sounds a little tough to never use the following words: no, couldn't, wouldn't, shouldn't, can't, never, not – to name a few. Instead I had to learn to tell the child "what to do," NOT "what not to do." My son is now 16 months and I treat him with this same respect, and the results are fabulous. Give it a try and while you are at it, try it with your spouse and adult friends. You may find that when you tell your husband to "remember the milk" rather than "don't forget the milk," you will actually get the milk.

Leslie, mother of Connor William, age 16 months
Ontario, Canada

At age 6 months your baby will start to respond to his/her name and also react to angry and friendly tones. He/She will also vocalize with intonation. By age 12 months your child may use one or more words and be familiar with the meaning. He/She will also be able to understand simple directions and imitate sounds. At age 18 months your baby will know between 5 to 20 words, mainly nouns. By 24 months your baby will be able to name objects, use prepositions, combine words, and use pronouns.

**Elaine Emily Dreyfuss, speech pathologist and mother of Emil, age 7
New Jersey**

Always listen to what is being said by your child. Also listen to what is not being said. You may learn more from what is left out than by what is included. Children are masters at rhetoric.

**Milynda, social worker and mother of Leif, age 16, and Mackinley, age 13
Michigan**

Have more than one tool in your mothering toolbox. Be a "positive" mother. Creatively avoid the use of negative words and actions (no, stop, don't, etc.) by being positive (let's try this, let's go outside, let's read, let's rock in the chair).

**Edna, high school teacher and mother of Sarah, age 23, and Allan, age 19
Texas**

One thing we have learned professionally and through personal experience is to use "Self Talk" and "Parallel Talk" as early as two months.

SELF TALK and PARALLEL TALK: Talk out loud about what you and/or your child are seeing, hearing, doing, or feeling when your child is nearby and within hearing range. He does not have to be close to you or pay attention to you when you talk out loud: he only has to be within hearing range. Be sure to use slow, clear, simple words and short phrases. Children learn speech from listening to others! For more information and suggestions, visit www.talkingchild.com.

Amy Chouinard, speech language pathologist and mother of Charlie, age 2 months, and Cory Poland, speech language pathologist and mother of Ally, age 2, and Ana, age 4 months

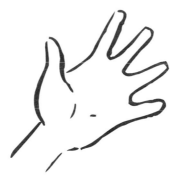

— Signing with Baby —

Sign language not only stimulates multiple parts of the brain, but it also bridges the gap of communication. It offers a way for children to express their wants even if they do not yet have the ability to speak. Research has shown that babies who use symbolic gestures or signs have larger vocabularies, understand more words, and engage in more sophisticated play than nonsigning babies. Parents are often concerned that their children won't learn to talk if they are taught sign language. On the contrary, research suggests that their first spoken words are usually words they had learned to sign. Simple sign language promotes talking. As children learn to speak more words, their use of sign language fades away. For more information on sign language, visit www.talkingchild.com.

Amy Chouinard, speech language pathologist and mother of Charlie, age 2 months, and Cory Poland, speech language pathologist and mother of Ally, age 2, and Ana, age 4 months

Learn and teach your baby basic sign language. There are several good books and videos on the market. Start at 6 to 9 months old and speak while you are making the signs. Begin with basic things like "eat," "drink," "more," and "all done." It is amazing how quickly your baby will pick up on this new language and be able to communicate his/her needs to you before learning to speak. It sure lowered the frustration level in our house. We use it now to quietly remind the children to mind their manners in public.

Andrea, mother of Zachary, age 4, and Joshua, age 3
Texas

I learned sign language to teach my son when he was 7 months old. By 9 months he was signing back to me. This has to be the most amazing gift a parent can give a child. It has enhanced our relationship and taught me respect for him in ways not imaginable…all by the time he was a year old.

Leslie, mother of Connor William, age 16 months
Ontario, Canada

By introducing some basic signs from American Sign Language, you can significantly reduce the frustration of communicating for you and your baby.

Terese, infant sign instructor and mother of a girl, age 4½, and boy, age 2
Alberta, Canada

Consider using sign language with your baby. It's easy and rewarding, and the benefits are innumerable. Just teaching a few signs, such as "eat," "more," and "help," will ease frustration, and teaching more will enable you to have a lot of insight into your baby's mind. I've signed with two of my children, and seeing them sign "more milk" sure beats deciphering their wails any day.

Monica Beyer, owner of www.signingbaby.com, and mother of
Dagan, age 8, Corbin, age 5, and Lauren, age 21 months
Missouri

Learn some American Sign Language (ASL) signs to use with your preverbal baby or toddler. Visit www.weecansign.com to learn how. We had great success using signs with our son, and he could communicate his needs, observations, and feelings long before he could speak! It was truly a gift to be able to reduce frustration and increase our communication skills!

Shannon, parent educator for Wee Can Sign and mother of
Eli, age 5 and signing since 11 months of age
Nevada

If you learn basic sign language, you and your baby can talk to each other at 6 months of age. To find a workshop, go to www.sign2me.com.

Trish, teacher of the deaf and mother of
Tim, age 18, Ingrid, age 9, and Hans, age 5
New York

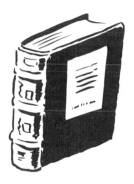

Teaching Baby

During my pregnancy I was working at a homeless shelter for teen moms and their kids, and I was always hitting the moms up for parenting advice, figuring if anyone knew the inside track on mama survival, it was them. One particularly conscientious and attached mom of a five-month-old advised me, "Don't hold your baby too much." I was a little surprised because of the hands-on parenting approach she used with her daughter, but she elaborated. "Hold your baby for playtime and when he's eating and definitely pick him up right away when he cries. But when he's happy, put him down as much as you can." She told me that when I experienced the magic of a tiny newborn in my arms, I would want to hold him endlessly. "If you do, he will expect to be held constantly until he is crawling, and it will make your life very challenging." I remember putting my three-week-old son down in his bouncy seat and struggling with the fact that, instinctually, I wanted him in my arms. But I followed the advice I'd been given, and it paid off in the form of an unbelievably mellow and independent baby who still loves lots of cuddles with his mama.

Sonya, social worker and mother of Luca, age 10 months
Minnesota

Help your child to learn and grow to the fullest potential; however, allow your child to enjoy being a child. (That does not mean to "baby" your child for an unnecessarily long time.)

Beverly, teacher and mother of three sons
Tennessee

Within reason, allow your children to try to do for themselves.

Beverly, teacher and mother of three sons
Tennessee

Our children come to help us grow. They are mirrors to us. They imitate what we say and how we act. They take on the essence of how we present ourselves in the world. I have often found that something my daughter is doing that I don't prefer came right from me in the first place. I can help her by improving myself.

Sherri, mother of Emma, age 3½
New York

Train your child to be honest. They learn from what they hear. Never talk in front of them about their misbehavior or they will think it is just as you say, "cute," and will repeat it until you find a satisfactory way to train them effectively. An infant is very well capable of learning a lot, so beware of what you may unintentionally teach them.

Phoebe, RN, LCCE, mother of Marie, age 37, Craig, age 34, Michelle, age 33, and Marsha, age 32, and grandmother of Gabriella, age 13, Matthias, age 10, Erik, age 7, James, age 7, Ethan, age 5, Alek, age 4, Caleb, age 18 months, Andrew, age 17 months, and Zachary, age 13 months
Tennessee

Don't be afraid to cuddle your baby for fear of spoiling him/her. Showing your baby affection creates a more secure, confident baby. Spoiling comes from not knowing when to say "no" at appropriate times. "Spoiling" and "loving" are really unrelated. Learn the difference and enjoy your baby full-heartedly as a parent should. All babies thrive on love!

Kathy, mother of Sophie, age 3
Nova Scotia, Canada

Older babies and toddlers find security in a daily schedule that's roughly the same each day. That way they know what to expect and can take comfort in the fact that they know what will happen next.

Heidi, courtesy of The Center for Conscious Parenting, www.cfcp.info, "run-outside-of-the-house" mom and mother of Heather, age 20 months
Oregon

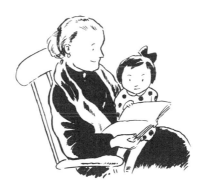

—Reading to Baby—

Books, books, books! Read to your children from the get go! I even read out loud while I was pregnant with my first. When I was pregnant with my second (my sons are 20 months apart), he, of course, heard me reading out loud to his older brother. I know I make plenty of mistakes as a mother, but the one thing I'm sure I'm doing right is instilling a love of books. Although my sons are now reading (my third grader reads well beyond his years), I still read to them every night. If we have a sitter, I insist that the sitter reads to them.

Monica McNeeley, actress and mother of Griffin, age 9, and Trent, age 7
Pennsylvania

If your young children want to hear the same story over and over again, don't worry about it. Children take comfort from the familiarity and predictability of a beloved story that they know by heart. There's no harm in that. Reread old favorites and, at the same time, introduce your children to new stories. Your children's minds and hearts have room for both.

Barbara Freedman-De Vito, author and artist at Baby Bird Productions Children's
Stories and Fairy Tales, www.babybirdproductions.com
Massachusetts

My biggest tip of all is books, books, books. Read to your child when you bring him/her home from the hospital, and your child will be an avid reader forever.

**Georgeanne, labor and postpartum doula and mother of four
and grandmother of four
Maryland**

It's never too early to begin reading to children. Start while your children are still in infancy. Let babies get familiar with the look and feel of books – have cloth or other soft books in the playpen. Read to babies, show them the pictures in the books, and sit them on your lap at the computer to see online pictures and animations. Let them hear the sounds of the words even when they're too young to understand them. Establish a positive association between the words and images on the printed page or computer screen and the warmth and security of mom's or dad's lap during a special quiet sharing time. Then read to them on a regular basis – throughout babyhood and toddlerhood and the preschool years and on up into elementary school. It's the best way to develop the good reading skills that will be so important for your children's success as they grow up. If you encourage your older children to read to your littler ones, it can also be a nice way to build strong relationships between your children.

**Barbara Freedman-De Vito, author and artist at Baby Bird Productions Children's
Stories and Fairy Tales, www.babybirdproductions.com
Massachusetts**

This is a recommended reading list for babies up to preschool age from the American Library Association.

Ten, Nine, Eight by Molly Bang; *Goodnight Moon* by Margaret Wise Brown; *Mike Mulligan and His Steam Shovel* by Virginia Burton; *The Very Hungry Caterpillar* by Eric Carle; *Julius the Baby of the World* by Kevin Henkes; *The Snowy Day* by Ezra Jack Keats; *If You Give a Mouse a Cookie* by Laura Numeroff and Felicia Bond; *My Very First Mother Goose* by Iona Opie/ Rosemary Wells; *The Tale of Peter Rabbit* by Beatrix Potter; *Read Aloud Rhymes for the Very Young* by Jack Prelutsky; and *"More, More, More," Said the Baby* by Vera Williams.

**Maryellen, senior art director and mother of
Matthew, age 20, and Kevin, age 19
Pennsylvania**

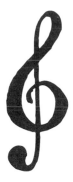

Encouraging Creativity

Creative thinking is essential for success in life, and it's our job as parents to nurture our kids' innate desire to be creative. By providing children with activities that use their creativity and imaginations, we are also giving them an important tool to deal with life down the road. Chances are, if you are a creative person, your child will be, too. You display creativity in your everyday activities like when you reason with a disgruntled child, change lyrics to songs, and maybe even do some interpretive dancing to entertain a toddler. It's a great idea to point out to your kids — no matter how young — how you use creativity in your daily life.

Susan Stump, owner of ChildCrafter Co., www.childcrafter.com, and mother of Kyle, age 2, and Alex, age 9 months
Pennsylvania

Provide a variety of brightly colored items in the baby's room to stimulate baby to explore. For the first few months, the baby is attuned to sight, smell, and sound. Introduce different scents to smell, colors and shapes for sight, and music for sound. Some types of music have been found to soothe even the crankiest of baby. And talk to your baby. It will teach your child the sound of your voice and give a sense of security.

Teresa Malone, freelance writer, owner of www.geocities.com/simple_variety (baby blankets and afghans), and stepmother
Kentucky

Visit museums and watch the performing arts. Surround your kids with culture. Expand their horizons with visual and performing arts. Maybe they'll start singing and dancing around your house.

Susan Stump, owner of ChildCrafter Co., www.childcrafter.com, and mother of Kyle, age 2, and Alex, age 9 months
Pennsylvania

Infants, toddlers and preschoolers are absorbing new information and learning all the time, so make the most of it. Stimulate their intellects and imaginations with storywriting, artwork, music, and dance. Provide them with a rich environment and let them test out any and all areas of creativity. That way, if they have some special talent in any field, it will have an opportunity to be discovered and nurtured; and, if not, your children will still be happier and more fulfilled for having had the chance to explore and experiment and find satisfying hobbies that suit their personalities and provide hours of lifelong pleasure. Be careful, however, never to push children into pursuing endeavors or sticking with activities that they have lost interest in. Creative arts should be fun, not stressful. Don't try to fulfill your own aspirations through your children; allow them the freedom to discover their own dreams and interests.

Barbara Freedman-De Vito, author and artist at Baby Bird Productions Children's Stories and Fairy Tales, www.babybirdproductions.com
Massachusetts

Babies love music. Introduce it to your baby early and don't feel limited to traditional "children's" music. Make it a part of your family life. We played music all the time for our son, even in the NICU. He responded well to the Beatles, show tunes, Vivaldi, lullabies, and the Gypsy Kings. Strangely, he did not like jazz. We took him to his first concert — Ray Charles — when he was just a few months old. He's three now and loves k.d. lang, Neil Young, Outkast, the *Jesus Christ Superstar* soundtrack, Simon and Garfunkle, Big Head Todd and the Monsters, Mr. Ray, Johnny Cash, Mummers music, the Beatles, and, yes, he still doesn't like jazz. We take him to outdoor concerts, and he has a blast dancing and clapping. We sing a lot in the car. The sweetest thing is that he sings and hums to himself as he plays. Music is a part of him and, like reading, will hopefully be a lifelong love.

Connie, publisher and mother of Holden, age 3
New Jersey

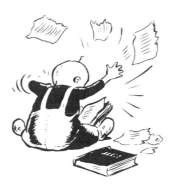

Discipline

Encourage your child to help out at an early age. They are just LOOKING for ways to please you and showing them simple chores (starting as soon as they can walk without holding onto something) will encourage good habits early. Not only has my son HAPPILY been throwing away his own dirty diapers for the past year and a half, he also puts his dirty clothes in his hamper, carries (unbreakable) dishes to the sink after a meal, turns off the TV at meal time, and throws away his trash. For example, I have discovered that when I encourage my son to turn off the television before a meal he will protest as he walks over to shut it off…but if *I* turn it off myself we have drama and chaos for ten minutes because he wants to watch TV and doesn't want to eat dinner. I have come to believe it's all in the presentation…

Kim, mother of Blake, age 3
California

Always try to see the world from your child's perspective. Ask yourself: If I were this child, how would I want my mother to respond? That question helps me respond appropriately to upsetting or frustrating situations.

Jennifer, stay-at-home mother of Milo, age 15 months
Illinois

At the very first La Leche League meeting I attended I heard the leader who was giving the speech say to her 2½ year old, "You don't want me to talk? But I need to talk. What can I do to make it work for both of us?" She went on to suggest several options; the toddler accepted a snack, and the mother went on with her talk. And I had just learned more in that exchange than I would learn from the mother's talk, which was excellent. What can I do to make it work for both of us? I think that little question lies at the heart of what child rearing is all about, and it's very important when it comes to discipline. First, we have to think about what it is we're trying to accomplish with our little ones. When it comes right down to it, we're not really raising children: we're raising adults. This means we're raising future employees, future managers, future husbands or wives, and future parents who all are going to live and work in an adult world that plays by adult rules. In the adult world, how do people ideally resolve their conflicts? With spankings? With time-outs? For the most part it's with conciliation, trying to come up with a solution where everyone is a winner. What do we need to do to make it work for all of us? At least that's how it should be. My job as a parent is not to rule over my child, making sure she "respects my authority" by obeying my every command. My job is to show her as she grows how she can get her needs and desires met while also taking into account the needs and desires of those around her. I first need to model this for her and meet her needs and desires in a way that works for me, too. For example, on a day that my need to get us out of the house quickly runs up against my daughter's need to nurse, I put her in a sling and let her nurse while I bustle about. Another example of a win-win situation that Laura and I came up with involved diapers. By 8 months Laura would vigorously protest being laid on her back for a diaper change. She would cry and wiggle and squirm, and it just wasn't working. Yet since she was not fully potty trained, I needed her to wear a diaper. What ended up working for us was that I switched her to training pants covered with rubber pants. I could/can now quickly change her while holding her in my arms, and it is no longer an ordeal. Laura very seldom protests a diaper change now. I have seriously read advice to make your baby "submit to the diaper change" by whatever means necessary under those circumstances. However, I believe the process Laura and I went through of finding a solution that works for both of us not only is easier on both our emotions, but more closely reflects how the world works in a good situation. This is the kind of situation I eventually want my daughter to be working in or the kind of marriage I want her to enjoy. She will be equipped to seek out and recognize such situations if that is what she learned at home.

Fernanda, mother of Laura, age 1
Colorado

If your child is "misbehaving," ask "What need does he/she have that is not being met right now?" Having a daily rhythm goes a long way in minimizing the need for discipline. When the child is in the flow of the day, he/she is less likely to act out.

Sherri, mother of Emma, age 3½
New York

When we baby-proofed our house, we put stick-on bumper pads on the edge of the coffee table. When our son started to pull himself up, he discovered he could pull the edging off the table. Nothing we could do would stop him. So, even though we had vowed not to spank or hit as discipline, I finally decided that slapping his hand was my only option. When I did it, he gave me such a look of stunned hurt that I immediately burst into tears. I realized that there were so many other things I could have tried – redirection being the most obvious. Since then, as I've learned more and watched him grow, I've come to see that my gut reaction (NOT to hit, in this case) is always the best. As a mother, you know your child intimately, and you know what's best for him/her. Trusting your instincts is always right, whether it's with your discipline, dealing with a doctor, grandparents, what have you. Seek out advice, sure, but don't discount yourself!

Melina, strategic workforce planning consultant and mother of Sebastian, age 2¾

Start as you mean to go on.

Davina, housewife and mother of Felix, age 7, Cecily, age 5, and Jemima, age 2

Babies know a LOT more than we give them credit for. Do not talk about their misbehavior in front of them except to THEM. They learn from what they hear, and it will not help you if you expose their bad behavior as "cute" to others. They are clever and can be a step ahead of us – be careful to be consistent in what you desire them to be. Do not threaten and then not produce. And never threaten severe punishment that you would never administer. This breeds mistrust!

Phoebe, RN, LCCE, mother of Marie, age 37, Craig, age 34, Michelle, age 33, and Marsha, age 32, and grandmother of Gabriella, age 13, Matthias, age 10, Erik, age 7, James, age 7, Ethan, age 5, Alek, age 4, Caleb, age 18 months, Andrew, age 17 months, and Zachary, age 13 months
Tennessee

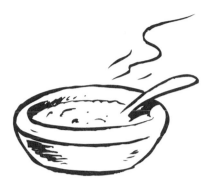

Introducing Solids

We waited until our twins were 7 months old to introduce solids. My yoga teacher explained how delicate their systems were and how simplicity was best. As a result, I breastfed and supplemented with fresh almond milk. When they turned 7 months old, I started introducing individually mashed avocado, mashed peas, carrots, baked apples, bananas, baked squash, and really easily digestible fruits and vegetables. Grains weren't introduced for a couple of months later. This way of eating helped prevent them from getting colds and being congested. So often you see babies and toddlers with runny noses or sounding congested. I think the best advice I ever received was to keep their diets very simple and don't be in such a rush to introduce such a wide variety of foods.

Victoria, film accountant and mother of twins, Jeff, Jr., and Diana, age 3
New York

When my daughter started on solid foods, I wanted her to eat healthy. Once a week, or even once every two weeks, I would steam up vegetables, mash them, put them in small jewelry baggies, and freeze them. You can also use small plastic cups with lids that restaurants use for dressing, etc. When it was time to eat, I popped them in the microwave and dinner was served! I also did this with meatloaf, ham, turkey, and chicken, but I cut them into very small pieces. My five-year-old still loves vegetables!

Kelly Taylor, founder of ProudParenting.com, and mother of Cameron, age 5

It is a myth that children love junk food. If you feed your children only healthy things, they will eat and enjoy healthy things. Don't feed them sugar! My 16-month-old's favorite meal is artichokes with pasta and sauce. She has had sugar only three times in her entire life, and there was a marked difference in her behavior each time. Read all labels and, if possible, make your children's food yourself.

Susan, mother of Athena, age 16 months
Colorado

Good eating habits start early. If at first you don't succeed…According to the American Academy of Pediatrics, many children will not accept a new food until it has been offered at least ten times. So if your child does not like some of the healthful foods you present…try, try again.

Tammy Pelstring, CEO, Obentec, Inc., creators of LapTop Lunches and mother of
Phoenix, age 10, and Triton, age 7
California

I fed my baby her baby food while I bathed her in the bathtub. I saved time, and the spilled food went right down the drain so I did not have to worry about the mess or clean up.

Kristi, therapist and mother of Zoe, age 15 months
Texas

After my girls were six months old, I made my own baby food. I would boil one onion, one potato, one yellow squash, a pinch of salt, a drizzle of oil, and either turkey breast or a fillet of tilapia and boil for about half an hour. Then I would process in a food processor and end up with some great tasting baby food. And, it lasts for three days in the refrigerator so you only have to make it about twice a week.

Cathy, nurse and mother of
Niki, age 3, Marina, age 1, and Baby # 3 due in April
New Jersey

I made my own baby food and froze the extra in ice cube trays – it's the perfect serving size.

Jessica, mother of Steven, age 6, Olivia, age 5, and George, age 2
New Jersey

I don't know how I didn't get the memo, but when my son was very small, I was told to give him juice, preferably apple juice, in his bottle. So I did. Unbeknownst to me, you are supposed to dilute with water by half to two-thirds before feeding! I also discovered…NEVER put the child in white when feeding him straight apple juice!

Deedy, mother of David
Oklahoma

It is best to introduce the vegetable baby foods before the fruit baby foods. This way your baby won't get accustomed to (and prefer) the sweetness of fruits. I started out with the vegetables with both of my children, and they both still love their vegetables, even spinach and brussels sprouts!

Tanya, stay-at-home mother of Dennis, age 5, and Joseph, age 1
Florida

Beware that by enabling or encouraging the child to eat only a few food items, the parent may be missing a prime opportunity to expand the diversity of the child's palate, taste preferences and food repertoire, all of which will have consequences later in life.

Parents might look to themselves in the face of a picky eater. Where might the child have picked up the idea that special accommodations around food represent acceptable behavior? Might the parent inadvertently be modeling such behaviors or eating attitudes at restaurants by asking for salads without dressing, fish hold-the-oil? Kids learn from what parents do, and do not do. They learn intentionally and unintentionally. They never stop watching and learning.

Abigail H. Natenshon, MA, LCSW, GCFP, author of *When Your Child Has an Eating Disorder: A Step-by-Step Workbook For Parents and Other Caregivers*, www.empoweredparents.com, and mother of two children
Illinois

Make a whole batch of food in the blender and freeze it in ice cube trays, small plastic containers, or (the easiest) ready-made containers specially designed for baby food storage. Nutritious food is ready whenever you need it – just thaw in a bowl of boiling water for 10 to15 minutes.

Dana Fleetham, www.naturalfamilyboutique.com and mother of Jubal, age 8, Calliope, age 5, Lydia, age 2, and Milo, age 7 months
Ohio

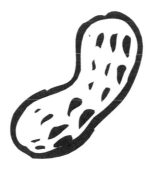

Allergies

The protein in cow's milk is one chemical that can set off an allergic reaction in some babies, affecting about 1 in 50 babies. Possible symptoms include skin reactions – hives or eczema – breathing difficulties, unsettled behavior, diarrhea, and vomiting. Medical attention should be sought if any of these occur. A baby is more likely to become allergic to something, including cow's milk, if a family member has asthma, hay fever, or any food allergies. If you think your child may have a cow's milk allergy, check with your doctor to be sure. Allergy testing these days is relatively painless and should be considered. Often babies who are allergic to cow's milk have allergies to other types of milk, such as soy and goat's milk.

From mothers of children who are volunteers of the Bonnie Babes Foundation
Victoria, Australia

Avoid dairy and nuts while breastfeeding. It passes into the milk, and if there is a predisposition to allergy, the baby can become sensitized to it. Allergists also say to avoid feeding your child peanut products (including peanut butter) until at least 4 years old. It seems that they are beginning to believe that the increase in peanut allergies is due to giving peanut butter and other peanut products at such an early age. Kids are becoming sensitized to it and that is causing the allergies. According to our doctor, if the child has other allergies or symptoms of allergies, then you should hold off until age 4. There is literature available online as well.

Debbie, owner of www.coconutbeach.com, and mother of
CJ, age 6½, and Rachel, age 2
New Jersey

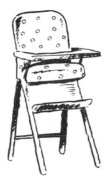

Self Feeding

As the mother of twin girls, I absolutely hated cleaning the high chairs and booster seats after every meal. As soon as my girls were old enough to sit without being strapped in, I ordered each of them one of the booster seats used in many restaurants. It is called a dual booster seat. It is the two-sided seat the offers a choice in heights so that they could sit at the dining table or flip it over and sit at the breakfast bar. Better yet, it is a one-piece molded unit that can be easily washed in the kitchen sink. It comes in many colors, including the basic beige that will go with any décor. You can order one from most restaurant supply stores. What a joy not to have to unstrap those ugly primary-colored seats anymore and get all the mess out from under them and out of every little crevice!

Debbie, full-time mother of twins Laura and Natalie, age 3
Alabama

The Neet Sheet has become a treasured friend in our household. I WAS a clean fanatic before and have learned that when my children started feeding themselves, by simply placing the sheet under the high chair, they could make a huge mess if they wanted to; and all I had to do was wash the sheet in the washing machine when they were done. This saved my carpet, my good towels, and most of all, my sanity.

Gina, banker and mother of Amanda, age 8, and Lilli, age 2
Florida

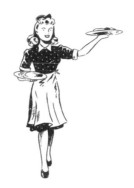

— Dining with Baby —

Before we take our baby out, we always feed him right before we go. Our children always seemed to get hungry while smelling the food, so if their tummies were full, they were more satisfied. Take in the baby carrier, but hold the baby while ordering and waiting for the food to arrive. This allows the baby not to become tired of the carrier. When your food arrives, place the baby in the carrier and hand him/her a rattle. This technique works wonders for keeping the baby occupied at the correct times.

**Kimberly, stay-at-home mother of
Haiden, age 9, Karsyn, age 5, and Nathan, age 6 months
Alabama**

Build a restaurant goodie bag of stickers and toys for your baby to keep her busy at the restaurant. There should be toys that she does not usually play with so they will be new and exciting at the restaurant. Always pack some plastic chain links (available in the infant section of almost any store) to hook onto the high chair to dangle the toys. That way you won't have to pick up toys over and over. Also try to get the kind of high chair that hooks to the table. These are great to take to restaurants because you don't have to worry about the germy high chairs they have, and the table high chairs can go to the park and almost anywhere. They are way better than booster seats because many times you don't have an extra chair to hook a booster seat to.

**Kristi, therapist and mother of Zoe, age 15 months
Texas**

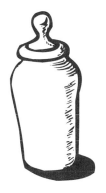

Weaning

Starting at six or seven months, introduce a cup. Put breast milk or formula in the cup, not only water. Too many kids think the bottle is only for milk and the cup is only for water, so they have a more difficult transition at a year when it is time to get rid of that bottle.

Jenny, Parents as Teachers educator and mother of Ben and Emma

Don't wean your baby until baby is ready; definitely not in the first year!

Morgan, mother of Kieran, age 17 months
New York

Putting water in the nighttime bottle once your child is "old enough" is a great way to give him/her the comfort wanted while not putting milk and sugar on his/her teeth just in time for bed.

Teresa, mother of Korinne, age 2

I started weaning my son at about 9 months by cutting out one nursing session and replacing with a bottle feeding. I gradually did this until we were down to the bedtime feeding. This one was hard — for both — to give up (probably harder on me than on him!). Finally at about 13 months, he was weaned. I was sad but grateful for the experience.

Connie, publisher and mother of Holden, age 3
New Jersey

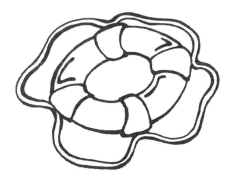

Life Savers

Always keep baby wipes handy! Even as your baby gets older and you don't need them for diaper changes, they are great for wiping hands at the playground, getting food off clothes, cleaning off the shopping cart, and pretty much anything! Kids are full of surprises!

**Jennifer, stay-at-home mother of
Karlie and Brooke, age 4, and Morgan and Emily, age 14 months**

Caller ID is sooo worth it! Those first few weeks when your rest is so important, Caller ID lets you decide who you talk to (and if the caller is just a pesky telemarketer!). It was a godsend for me with my first and a double godsend with my second!

**Jennifer, marketing manager and mother of
Will, age 2½, and Mary Catherine, age 14 months
Virginia**

I always layer five crib sheets and pads in the crib so I don't have to change the crib if it gets wet in the middle of the night. I just pull off one sheet and pad, and there is another set ready to go.

**Julie, mother of Connor, age 4, Carter, age 2, and Tyler, age 2 months
Indiana**

My second child was extremely fussy unless he was being held. With a busy 3-year-old also, I was having a hard time getting things done. A friend of mine recommended a sling. For the next months, the sling turned out to be one of the best ways to calm my fussy baby. It also provided privacy for nursing in public. When he was 6 months old and over 20 pounds, it also provided my back with the added support it needed. He is now two and still happy to be carried in his sling. It works great in those times when a stroller is not appropriate but I don't want him mobile.

Beth, lactation consultant and mother of
Ryan, age 5, and Jack, age 2
Pennsylvania

To remove crayon marks from walls, use WD-40.

Susan Gmeiner, president of Maya Wrap and mother of
Arj, age 14, Michael, age 12, and Karl, age 4
North Carolina

You will need your hands free all the time for burping, feeding, changing, cooking, etc., so buy a headset to plug into your phone. That way you can talk and keep up with all your tasks. Many times you'll need the supportive friend phone call, or it could be any other type of call that you need to take, yet can't stop what you are doing!

Christine, mother in constant training and mother of
Julia, age 2½, and Olivia, age 6 months
New Jersey

For convenience of changing the crib mattress sheet, NoJo brand makes a pad that you tie on to the crib slats and on top of the sheet. When baby drools, etc., you just untie and wash the pad instead of replacing the sheet which is back breaking after holding baby all day.

Another tip is to invest in a Roomba vacuum. My toddler throws food all over my clean house and instead of stressing, I just sit and read him a book while the Roomba does all the work for us! He now turns it on himself. The only thing is that it makes you lazy, and you can pack on the pounds by not actually doing the labor of vacuuming.

Angela, homemaker and mother of Dylan, age 10, and Nicholas, age 1½
California

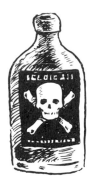

Safety Concerns

I do not use any chemicals in my household — not even dish detergent. Vinegar can clean just about anything that any chemical can without leaving a chemical residue on countertops and the like to be picked up by the next item you make to eat or the floor where your baby's toys sit and then go into his/her mouth. It's very simple to fill a couple of spray bottles with plain vinegar. Whenever there's a mess, I use that. You could also add some essential oils to help with cleaning, and there are some great books available with recipes for clothing detergents, dish detergents, floor cleaners, and so on.

But simple vinegar is so easy and costs less than any chemical cleaner. The smell dissipates immediately once it dries. I even mop the floor with it.

Diana, homemaker and mother of Logan, age 3, and Anika, age 3 months
New Jersey

Safe guard everything. Keep cleaning supplies and other toxic chemicals in upper cabinets or locked cabinets. Include medicines and makeup in this category also. Place covers over electrical outlets and secure cords. Put fasteners on cabinets and drawers. (These can be found at hardware stores.)

Teresa Malone, freelance writer, owner of www.geocities.com/simple_variety
(baby blankets and afghans), and stepmother
Kentucky

Keep your head in an emergency. Know the symptoms and have a plan (choking, falls, etc.). Don't panic in front of your child because that will cause your child to panic. Your child does not need to be any more scared than he/she already is. It is much more comforting if a parent is clearheaded, comforting, and is taking charge of the situation. Take all head injuries seriously. Always check the child's eyes for proper pupil dilation, even if he/she didn't lose consciousness. If your child is nauseous or vomiting following a head injury, follow up immediately with a doctor/hospital. Again, know the symptoms. It's always better to be safe than very sorry.

**Debbie, owner of www.coconutbeach.com, and mother of
CJ, age 6½, and Rachel, age 2
New Jersey**

Follow these tips from Kids in Danger to prevent injuries in strollers.

1. Follow the manufacturer's instructions on assembly, care, and use.

2. Ensure that latches are fully engaged prior to use. Injuries occur when strollers appear to be fully set up yet collapse when they hit a bump.

3. Don't overload the stroller — it may cause it to tip.

4. Always use restraints in the manufacturer's recommended use position. When using a carriage or a stroller in a fully reclined position for an infant, make sure there are no openings a child could slip fully or partially through.

5. Never leave a child unattended in a stroller — it is not a safe environment for sleeping or playing.

6. When folding or unfolding a stroller, please keep children away to avoid pinched fingers.

According to the U.S. Consumer Product Safety Commission (CPSC), over 11,000 children are rushed to emergency rooms each year from injuries related to strollers. Carriers and car seats are the only juvenile products responsible for more injuries. The CPSC lists recalled products from baby monitors to toys for the bathtub on their Web site, www.cpsc.gov. Do not use products if they have been recalled. Contact www.KidsinDanger.org, the manufacturer, or CPSC at 800-638-2772 to find out how to comply with recalls. Be sure to return product registration cards so that the manufacturer can contact you directly in case of a recall.

**Nancy, child safety advocate and mother of Hannah, Lucy, and Walter
Illinois**

When your baby can sit up, bathe him/her in the bathtub in a laundry basket. He/She won't fall over, and toys are within easy reach!

**Ronni , nurse midwife and mother of Isaac, age 4, and Emmett, age 2
Pennsylvania**

Children are especially vulnerable to pesticides' effects because, pound for pound, children eat more food, drink more water, and breathe more air than adults. For example, infants under age 1 consume 15 times more apple products relative to their body weight than the national average, yet apples have the highest pesticide residues of any fruit. Children's immature metabolic systems are also less able to detoxify and excrete many chemical toxins. Plus, children have a greater relative exposure to harmful substances because they crawl, play outside, and put things in their mouths more than adults do. In studying eight different pesticides, the National Resources Defense Council found that, on average, preschoolers received four times greater exposure to harmful pesticides than adults.

That's why it makes good sense to be cautious with food, one of the primary sources of exposure to pesticides for most children. Apples, pears, peaches, and grapes are among the most common sources of exposure for American children age 5 and under, according to a recent analysis of federal data by the Environmental Working Group (EWG).

While no food will ever be completely pesticide-free due to the environmental persistence of these chemicals, choosing organic food can dramatically reduce a child's exposure. In 2002, the first scientific comparison of organic and conventionally grown produce found that organic fruits and vegetables do indeed contain fewer pesticide residues overall. A 2003 study from the University of Washington also found that preschool children who ate organic food had one-sixth the concentration of pesticides in their bodies as did children who ate conventionally grown food. In the study, children who ate organic food had pesticide exposure levels below EPA safety standards, while the children on conventional diets tested above those standards.

Even if you can't get organic fruits and vegetables, you can still reduce pesticide exposure. Certain conventionally grown fruits and vegetables such as blueberries and broccoli are naturally lower in pesticide residues than other conventionally grown produce.

Rochelle Davis, Excerpt from *Fresh Choices: More Than 100 Easy Recipes for Pure Food When You Can't Buy 100% Organic* by David Joachim and Rochelle Davis
Rodale Books, 2004
Illinois

There is nothing more precious than the well-being of your children. It is crucial to perform in-depth background checks on each person working in your home or/and with your children. If you do not feel qualified to screen your employees, an agency is most always available to assist you.

Amy Brixey, owner of The Nanny Option and mother of Kellen, age 16 months
Missouri

Block off the kitchen with a baby gate, especially while cooking or baking. That way, you don't need to worry that your baby will touch the hot oven or pull something unsafe off the counters.

Kelly, babyproofer, owner of www.totsafe.com, and mother of Adam, age 3
Michigan

I did not write this (it is from babycenter.com), but I think it's important. Until August 1999, the American Academy of Pediatrics recommended against using any type of sunscreen on babies younger than 6 months. Their skin's ability to metabolize and excrete chemicals may not be fully developed. But the AAP now says that no evidence shows that using sunscreen on small areas of a baby's skin is harmful, and it's probably safe to use sunscreen on babies under 6 months if adequate clothing and shade aren't available. That doesn't mean you should slather your baby in sunblock, though. Just apply small amounts of lotion to the face and the back of hands. For all babies, the AAP recommends using brimmed hats and waterproof sunscreen. The AAP and American Academy of Dermatology recommend an SPF of at least 15, but many experts recommend 30 or higher for babies, and baby sunscreen formulas often have even higher SPF's. Apply sunscreen at least 20 minutes before sun exposure for it to seep in and reapply it after your baby has played in the water, even if it's waterproof.

Melissa, mother of
Harrison, age 3, Cade, age 2, and Nica, age 3 months

We all feel very rushed as mothers: the diaper needs to be changed NOW; the baby needs to be fed NOW; my child is whining and needs my attention NOW. You know what? You need to pay attention to yourself NOW. We give up a lot to raise these little beings who communicate mostly through crying, and it's stressful. Take everything you can at a pace you can handle. Don't rush to warm the bottle or hurry through the shower to pay more attention to Junior. You need attention, too. And mistakes and accidents are much more likely to occur when you are, say, running through the bathroom slipping on a wet floor as you rush to get your baby rediapered. A relaxed mom makes for relaxed babies. Take your time. Nothing can be that important.

Jennifer, part-time director of community relations and mother of
Grace, age 3½, and Anna, age 10 months
Iowa

Purchase these before the baby is born, even though most cannot be given until 6 months of age or are only for special circumstances. You won't believe how quickly 6 months goes by, and when you need these things, you need them immediately! Your baby will be feeling lousy (translate as "crying loudly and inconsolably"), and you won't want to run out to the drug store. It helps to have these all in one basket that you can grab and sort through easily. Some of these items you will want in each of your diapering stations (e.g., Mylecon, if your baby struggles with gas pains, etc.)

1. Infant Advil

2. Infant Tylenol (Yes, buy both. They have different purposes, durations of pain relief, etc.)

3. Infant Tylenol Cold

4. Baby Benedryl — often the first thing the nurses will tell you to give a a child when they suspect an allergic reaction to something

5. Mylecon Gas Drops

6. Ipecac syrup

7. Johnson Soothing Vapor Cream or Vapor Patches to help keep stuffy noses clear

8. Vaporizer (cool mist) — helps both for dry winter air and to create soothing white noise during naps/bedtimes

9. Liquid Vicks to put into the vaporizer for colds

10. Suction bulb for yucky noses (Babies love this.)

11. Ayr Nasal Saline or other saline drop for crusty noses — spray into nose and then suction out with suction bulb (They love this even more.)

12. Avent baby massage gel or lotion (Massage your baby! Newborns love this, and soon they are too squirmy to put up with this wonderful bonding activity between parent and child.)

13. Eucerin lotion – for all over moisturizing after bath

14. Cetaphil soap and lotion for sensitive skin — helps a lot with baby acne (Whatever you do, and no matter how tempted you are by your own memories of adolescence — don't pick!)

15. Hand sanitizing lotion – keep it everywhere

16. Rectal thermometer or good-quality ear thermometer

17. Nail clippers and baby Q-tips

18. Baby brush and comb

19. Travel kit for baby's first road trip with travel sizes of many of the items mentioned

**The contributing moms of "The List," a growing list
of new mom tips passed from friend to friend
New Jersey, Maryland, and Delaware**

The First Birthday

Realize that baby's first birthday party is more for you as a parent than it is for your child. Resist the urge to go overboard and plan something simple that won't overwhelm your child.

Kim Danger, owner www.mommysavers.com, and mother of
Sydney, age 5, and Nicholas, age 1
Minnesota

Your baby won't remember his/her first birthday party, so if you want to throw a big party, remember it's more about you than baby and plan accordingly. If mostly adults will be attending, don't be afraid to have an adult theme and food. If you have a lot of other babies or young children coming, make sure you have age-appropriate activities for them. Plan the party around your baby's best time of day, whether that's before or after his/her nap. Do something special to commemorate the day. I did a time capsule. Each guest was asked to bring something from the year my son was born. We had a little ceremony as everyone placed their objects in a large box. We also placed the invitation, pictures from my son's first year, pictures of our family, and a video from the party in the box. We'll open the time capsule when he is 18. We did the same thing for our daughter's first birthday. I think they will appreciate seeing these "treasures" when they are older.

Anonymous, teacher and mother of Michael, age 4, and Emily, age 1½
Maine

Your First Year

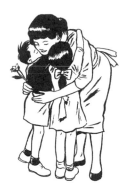

— Introducing Siblings —

Sibling rivalry has more to do with your relationship with your children than your children's relationships with one another. After all, for what are they rivaling? Primarily, their parents' attention or approval. Using this valuable insight, I've had ten children and NO "sibling rivalry." I DON'T let the new baby be an excuse for not spending time with them. I let them help when the new baby comes as far as I think their ability will let them but not so much that they come to view the baby as a burden. Don't let the older children feel sorry for themselves when the new baby arrives. Finally, you may have to trim your schedule of outside commitments for a few months to cement positive attitudes concerning your home. If your husband or any of the children feel less important than your outside commitments, you may need to reprioritize. It's such a short time in the big scheme of things, and the rewards are far greater than any other promise.

Susan, mother of Rebecca, age 17, Catherine, age 15, Philip, age 12, Paul, age 11, Marybeth, age 9, Hannah, age 8, Matthew, age 6, Mark, age 4, Joshua, age 3, and Joann, age 11 months
Texas

I have a 6-year-old stepson and an 8-month-old baby. When the baby was born, we made a note of telling guests to focus the first few minutes of their visit on the 6-year-old. This helped us control jealousy and after a few minutes, the big brother was ready to show off the baby!

Julie, purchasing manager, Chinaberry Inc., www.chinaberry.com, and mother of two
California

When you bring a new baby home from the hospital, don't expect your older child to share his things with the baby. He's already sharing his most important possessions – his parents! Don't make him share anything else in the beginning. Would you like it if your husband said, "Honey, I love having a wife so much, I'm going to get another one! She's going to be cute and get a lot of attention, and, by the way, please share your clothes and your kitchen with her." I don't think so! It makes the adjustment so much easier if you put yourself in your older child's shoes and are easy on him in the beginning in terms of sharing with the baby. This way you can try to avoid feelings of jealousy and resentment from the beginning.

Shosh, mother of Akiva, age 21 months, and Donny, age 6 months
Illinois

Each time I had a new baby, I made sure that my other children always felt included in everything I did. They helped feed the baby, change, and even give baths. On the day I came home with our new baby, I also gave each one of my daughters a new doll of her very own. To this day, there has never been any jealousy between the daughters. And I have also made it a point to never "label" them as being the oldest, middle, or baby of the family.

Denise, music teacher and mother of Carina, age 7, Cecilia, age 5, and Isabella, age 1
California

Have the baby and older sibling exchange gifts the first time they "meet." The older sibling will enjoy picking out a gift for his/her new baby brother or sister and will appreciate receiving a gift at a time when much of the focus is on the new arrival.

Moira Campbell, HypnoBirthing practitioner and mother of
Calum, age 5, and Isobel, age 2
British Columbia, Canada

When we first brought home our second child, we were understandably concerned about our 3-year-old's feelings. As soon as we got home, we had a little photo session. With my husband by my side, new baby in one arm and the other arm around my 3-year-old, my mother-in-law snapped the digital picture that saved us. My son saw the picture and proclaimed that mommy could hold both kids (and love them both!). And so I have. We still spend lots of time all sitting together.

Ann, mother of Billy, age 3, and Macy, age 1
Florida

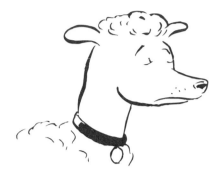

Introducing Pets

No matter how much you plan ahead, the addition of a new baby may be difficult for your pet. Remember, your dog or cat was your first "baby" and is used to being the center of your attention. So it's understandable that she may experience something akin to sibling rivalry when you introduce a new human baby into your household. You can minimize this feeling by working with her *before* you bring home your baby. For example, because your new baby will demand a lot of your time and energy, gradually accustom your pet to spending less time with you. Drastically decreasing attention and frequently scolding, ignoring, or isolating your pet *after* the baby comes home will likely make your pet feel stressed. If your pet is particularly attached to the mother-to-be, another family member should develop a closer relationship with the animal. That way, your pet can still feel loved and provided for while mom is busy with the baby.

Martha Jones, editor of www.therealmartha.com
Missouri

Before you bring your baby home from the hospital, have your partner or friend take home something with the baby's scent (such as a blanket) for your pet to investigate. When you return from the hospital, your pet may be eager to greet you and receive your attention. Have someone else take the baby into another room while you give your pet a warm, but calm, welcome. Keep some treats handy so you can distract your pet. After the initial greeting, you can bring your pet with you to sit next to the baby; reward your pet with treats for appropriate behavior. Remember, you want your pet to view associating with the baby as a positive experience. To prevent anxiety or injury, never force your pet to get near the baby, and always supervise any interaction. Try to maintain regular routines as much as possible to help your pet adjust. And be sure to spend one-on-one quality time with your pet each day—it may help relax you, too. With proper training, supervision, and adjustments, you, your new baby, and your pet should be able to live together safely and happily as one (now larger) family.

Martha Jones, editor of www.therealmartha.com
Missouri

It's easy for parents and grandparents to lavish so much time and attention on the new baby that other members of the household feel rejected and resentful. While we all know the importance of setting aside special times and activities that are just for you and each of your older children, it's easy to forget about the family pets. They, too, are trying to adapt to a new situation; so to help them accept the new arrival, you should try to give them the same level of affection and attention that they were already accustomed to receiving. Stick to the comfort of old routines as well, such as habitual feeding times and dog-walking schedules. These measures will make pets feel happier and more secure and thus will reduce the possibility of jealousy or negative behavior directed towards the baby.

With a new baby in the house, don't ban pets from the room or suddenly exclude them from family activities, but do supervise their interactions with the baby to ensure that jealousy or confusion over changes in the household don't manifest themselves in antisocial behavior. Use your own judgment, based on your knowledge of your pets and their responses to new situations, to help them learn to love the baby. By the same token, babies and young children need to be taught to be thoughtful and gentle when they are around pets. Teach them not to pull tails or handle animals roughly or frighten them with loud noises or sudden movements. Help your children to grow up respecting and caring about the welfare of their fellow creatures and enjoying their companionship. As your children mature they can also learn to be caring and responsible pet owners, a lesson which will help them to become more responsible human beings in general.

Barbara Freedman-De Vito, author and artist at Baby Bird Productions Children's
Stories and Fairy Tales, www.babybirdproductions.com
Massachusetts

Your First Days

Use the basic principles of time management to make those first days with baby as stress-free as possible by screening phone calls, limiting visitors, and putting the final touches on baby announcements. Delegate the task of announcing the birth of your baby to a family member or friend. If you did your homework during the pregnancy, you created a simple Web page to spread the word about your good news. Now all that's left to do is fill in the vital statistics (name, date of birth, height, and weight) to announce your exciting news to the world. Screen your phone calls and announce your baby's birth at the same time. Record a brief message on your voicemail or answering machine to provide friends and family with important information about baby, mom, and dad. Not only does it keep you from repeating yourself, but it also gives your household a much-needed break from visitors and allows you to settle into your new schedule.

**Debbie Williams, organizing strategist, www.organizedtimes.com, and mother of David, age 8,
Texas**

This is from a midwife I met. After the baby is born, mom should be expected to enjoy her babymoon and not be trying to overdo it. So mom should spend five days in bed, five days on bed, and then five days around bed. Wise words to live by – we try to cram so much in the first few weeks, and all we really need to do is get to know the new little person in our lives.

**Zoe, public health nurse, midwifery student, and mother of Vivian, age 2
Ontario, Canada**

Don't assume that you can automatically pick up where you left off before your baby was born. Employers typically give 6 to 8 weeks postpartum leave. Not that you should let your house and family "go to pot," but take some time before baby is born to prioritize your postpartum time. As a mother of nine, I overestimated my abilities when my 10th baby was born. Things were going well when she was four or five days old, so I started the other children back on their typical daily schedules (including homeschooling). As I reentered into my "work world," I could literally feel changes in my body. When my loving husband asked what (in the world!) I was doing going "back to work," we only talked for about 15 minutes before I decided that taking off for three or four weeks would be best for everyone. Immediately, I felt my body revert back to its recovering stage and milk let down for my baby girl to nurse. Unfortunately, I didn't understand this phenomenon with my 7th, 8th, and 9th babies and nursing them was progressively worse with each one until the 9th when I never really made enough milk to nourish him. RELAX and ENJOY YOUR FAMILY!

Susan, homemaker and mother of Rebecca, age 17, Catherine, age 15, Philip, age 12, Paul, age 11, Marybeth, age 10, Hannah, age 8, Matthew, age 6, Mark, age 5, Joshua, age 3, and Joann, age 11 months
Texas

Rest. I mean, *really rest*. Take care of yourself so you can take care of your baby. Put your feet up during feedings. Take some deep breaths. When the baby sleeps, take a nap or lie down. The first few weeks are a huge time of healing for your body. Don't push it. Take care of yourself — plan a rest time once a week even if it is only for a couple of hours. Nap when the baby naps — don't use that time for busy work. Learn to do your chores with baby in tow (they like watching you work – it's stimulating for them).

Elisabeth K. Corcoran, author of *Calm in my Chaos: Encouragement for a Mom's Weary Soul* (Kregel Publications, www.kregel.com), and mother to Sarah, age 7½, and Jack, age 6
Illinois

If you have a nonemergency question, you can always call the postpartum floor (that you were discharged home from) for advice on yourself, breastfeeding, or baby care. The nurses are up and available 24/7.

Dolores, R.N., Lamaze (LCCE), doula, and mother of
Jonathon and Megan
New York

Whilst baby naps during the day, use this time to catch up on sleep! And don't try to be a super mum!

Stacey, nanny and mother of Matthew, age 5 months
London, England

Those first few weeks are VERY difficult – you're tired, the baby never seems tired at the right time, you're overwhelmed. But as you lay there exhausted, dirty, and tired on the bed, staring at this new life, you can't believe how much you love this child. Yes, you love your husband, but this baby has just taught you the true meaning of the word love.

Jennifer, educator and mother of Samuel, age 12, Michael, age 7, and Emily, age 4
New Jersey

Rest, rest, rest! Okay, it sounds trite, and while pregnant, you've probably heard everyone in the world tell you to rest; but once you've given birth, it's even more important that you still adhere to the resting phase the first few days you are home from the hospital. I can't even begin to explain how much rest is needed after a cesarean section…but in either type of delivery, your body needs time to recuperate, so take it easy. What does resting mean? It could mean using paper plates so there are fewer dishes to wash. It could also mean having a friend or relative come sit with you a few hours a day and help you around the house (which is especially helpful if you have other younger children). And if you have older children, it could mean having them help out with more chores around the house. Most of all, it means to just let some things go. The dusting doesn't have to be done right away…perhaps it can wait a few more days, or weeks even.

Demetria Zinga, Web designer, freelance writer, and stay-at-home mother of
Nyomi, age 2
Alabama

As a new mother, you need to sleep when your baby sleeps. Although you may want to use that time to "catch-up" on household chores – DON'T! You are better off resting for your peace of mind and sanity. Rest, girl! You deserve and need it.

Cindy, mother of Caeley, age 6, and Cameron, age 4
California

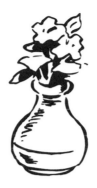

Visitors

When the baby comes home, don't invite everyone over. Take a week to get to know each other. Dad, Mom, and baby need to get to know each other without a crowd. If it's the first baby in the family, then schedule times when no one is there so all three of you can cuddle together. When I had my second and third children, we didn't invite anyone over for a week. It was quiet and wonderful.

Rosa, yoga studio owner and mother of
Paulina, age 13, Daniela, age 10, and Julia, age 9
Florida

I put a sign on my door during nap/quiet time. It simply said, "Please do not ring the bell. We are napping and will be out to play later."

Dawn, mother of Elizabeth, age 9, Tabitha, age 8, William, age 5, and Abigail, age 1
Virginia

New moms tend to be very territorial and overly conscientious about who is handling their baby and how their baby is being handled. I learned the hard way – especially after a C-section – that it is essential to accept help offered from friends and family during the first few weeks, and even months, so that a new mom can get her rest and recover. Don't try to do it ALL…prioritize and focus on getting your health back so that you can be ready to be a good mom!

Mary, financial services and mother of Lauren, age 13 months
Texas

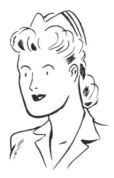

Accepting Help

Nighttime help is great. Use it if you can, especially if you are bottle feeding or pumping. Just a few extra hours sleep can help you be a better person — and a better mom — the next day.

Dr. Ruth Peters, clinical psychologist, author, "Today Show" contributor, and mother of Lindsay, age 25, and Chris, age 21
Florida

Learn to accept help! So many people offer assistance when you bring a new baby home, but it's easy to try and be polite and wave off any assistance because you want to be a supermom. But the fact is, the first few weeks can be overwhelming taking care of an infant, and mom's health can suffer. Your mother, mother-in-law, and mommy friends are all offering to help you because they know what you're going through. Allow friends to bring you meals, help fold the laundry, or babysit older siblings. Take everyone up on their offers and use the extra time to take care of you and your little one.

Shelly Drouin, StrollerFit instructor and mother of Haley, age 21 months
Texas

If someone volunteers to help – get it in writing.

Robbie, mother of Holl, age 2
Texas

Don't be afraid to ask for help. Ask everyone you know if you need to. A new mother needs as much support as she can get. Remember that we all have been in the same position you are, and we all needed some guidance at one time or another.

Kristin, teacher and mother of Lillian, age 2½
Pennsylvania

Hiring a baby nurse was the best thing we did! Our nurse was a wonderful, kind, experienced woman who was an expert in baby care because that's all she does – care for newborns. We didn't have to worry about not knowing how to do anything – we had a 24/7 consultant on hand to train us in "best practices." I wouldn't hesitate for a second to use a baby nurse again.

Elisa, management consultant and mother of Quinn, age 17 months
Colorado

The more help you can get, the better mom you'll be. Bonding does not have to occur in the first few days. It doesn't have to be all you. Share the burden and the pleasure. Your baby's psyche won't be damaged if your partner, mom, or baby nurse helps out. Remember — your baby won't even remember the first weeks!

Dr. Ruth Peters, clinical psychologist, author, "Today Show" contributor,
and mother of Lindsay, age 25, and Chris, age 21
Florida

Hire a postpartum doula. The postpartum doula can be a wonderful ally for breastfeeding. The support of a postpartum doula includes knowledgeable guidance regarding breastfeeding, newborn well-being, and your own postpartum concerns. Plus, a doula offers practical assistance with meal preparation, laundry, errands, and more. The model of care allows mothers to be cared for while they gain confidence and focus on the relationship with their newborn. It's not just the direct guidance with nursing that helps new mothers get off to a great start with breastfeeding. Another perk: the postpartum doula is with your family for at least a four-hour shift. If you are having challenges and need feedback on your nursing sessions, the doula will be witnessing multiple feedings, thereby collecting valuable information for you and your lactation consultant.

Karen Laing, lactation consultant, owner of Birthways Doula Services in Chicago, and
mother of Birkleigh, age 9 months
Illinois

Don't be afraid to ask for help. New parents are overwhelmed, functioning with limited sleep and slow-thinking brains. As relatives and neighbors volunteer to help with light housekeeping, cooking, or babysitting while you nap, take them up on their offer. As parents themselves, they know just what you are going through and are happy to help lighten your load. As friends, they are excited to spend time with your new baby and get to know him/her. And as family, they share the joy of welcoming another member into the fold, to love and nourish him/her as only loved ones do.

Debbie Williams, organizing strategist, www.organizedtimes.com, and mother of David, age 8,
Texas

For a few weeks before my due date, I cooked double batches of many favorites and froze them, and that helped me manage. However, when my last baby was 11 days old, I was readmitted to the hospital with a heart problem. Friends delivered hot meals to my front door for a month. Whenever anybody asked me what they could do to help, I asked for dinner. I also learned that it is OK to ask for something you need when you need it and that people were glad when I asked them to do a specific job.

Thesesa, stay-at-home mother of Bianca, age 25, Mary Catherine, age 20, Jon, age 16, Matt, age 13, Kevin, age 4
New Jersey

Accept every offer of help you get in those first few months – and always! Surround yourself with support. If your family isn't around (or even if they are, they may drive you crazy!) or your friends "just don't get it," a mothers' group like The Moms Club or Mothers and More can do wonders for you!

Sarah Zeldman, Life Balance coach – Balanced Woman Coaching,
www. Balanced-woman-coaching.com,
and mother of Yosef, age 3½, and Shanya, age 1
New York

Don't give up! Get professional help and support. Call a doula in your area for support and good local resources. Research Dr. Jack Newman's book/Web site.

Andrea, doula and mother of Christina, age 8
Canada

For all the expectant moms who do not have any relatives nearby, who are uncomfortable letting someone else care for your newborn as soon as you return from the hospital, or who are expecting multiples and need an extra pair of hands: consider looking into the value of having a baby nurse or postpartum doula come to your home to help you those first few weeks. Having one can cut back on your chances of postpartum depression, answer your newborn questions, get immediate help with breastfeeding, provide night care, and prepare meals for the family. That way you can truly get the much needed rest a new mom needs without worrying about what's not being done while you are recovering. Your recovery and peace of mind is so important in order to heal properly.

Valerie Ybarra, baby nurse, postpartum doula, owner www.baynurseonthego.com, and mother of Alexis, age 15, and Arianna, age 8
Georgia

Bringing your precious little one into this world is an incredible experience, and hiring a baby nurse to take care of your baby in the first few days of baby's life is one of the most important decisions you will ever make.

There are two categories of baby nurses: those who are certified and those who are not certified. Baby nurses with certification will have an educational background in pediatric nursing, early childhood development, or have a medical background that enables them to professionally care for a newborn. The rates for these professionals are usually very high, and they are normally hired when the baby/babies is/are born premature or have a medical condition. Noncertified baby nurses, however, usually gain their experience by hands-on care. Many of these professionals have extensive experience caring for no less than 15 newborns in one year. In my professional experience, I have observed that parents hire the noncertified baby nurses who have accumulated their experience over time, taking on one assignment after another, making them masters in the art of caring for newborns. They are usually contracted for a minimum of 14 days, which gives the exhausted new mom enough time to recuperate after giving birth. For normal, healthy babies, these noncertified baby nurses work great. But no matter which category of baby nurse you choose to hire, nothing beats a pair of professional, loving, caring, gentle hands, which usually comes in the form of great job references. So my advice to you when hiring is to look for a pair of professional, loving, caring, gentle hands! They always work.

Pauline Guy, owner Celebrities Staffing Services
California and New York

After the birth, have people sign up for certain days to cook a meal for the whole family. This is a great shower gift: someone prepares a list of names and then calls everyone after the birth, and meals are brought nightly for 2 to 3 weeks. It is necessary to rest a lot and to be with the baby in the beginning, not in the kitchen and standing for long periods of time.

Diane Hynes, shiatsu/craniosacral practitioner and mother of
Taegan, age 28 months
New Jersey

If finances allow, hire a doula and/or a cleaning service and let friends and family just do the cooking. If finances do not allow, be creative about how to get help. USE your friends and then do the same for them when they are new parents. Take out a loan to finance these expenses the way you would for a house or car. Being "extravagant" at this time will reap you and your partner more emotional and health rewards than a car or house ever will. Treasure this time in your baby's life and in your family life. It will be over in an instant, and it will never come again.

Meladee, courtesy of The Center for Conscious Parenting, www.cfcp.info, teacher
who is currently a very happy stay-at-home mother of Colin, age 5½,
and Rory, age 11 months
Oregon

When you become a mom for the first time, you must remember there is no perfect mother. Don't worry about the wash or the cleaning — it will all the there when you are ready. Take the time to get to know your new baby. Time moves so fast – enjoy every minute. When family and friends want to help, assign them those jobs of helping with the laundry and housework.

Dawn, RN, and mother of Sophia, age 3, and Analiese, age 1
New Jersey

Allow other people to pamper you. And if someone offers to help, actually give them something little to do. During baby's fussy times, find a friend or family member or husband to give you some relief for even an hour or so a day. Getting away from the screaming helps to handle it better.

Elisabeth K. Corcoran, author of *Calm in my Chaos: Encouragement for a Mom's Weary Soul*
(Kregel Publications, www.kregel.com), and mother to Sarah, age 7½, and Jack, age 6
Illinois

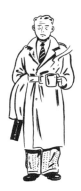

Your Partner

Even if you're breastfeeding, or maybe especially if you're breastfeeding, express and store enough milk for one feeding each day. Agree with Dad that he will get up once each night to feed baby. Dad gets to share those marvelous, quite, intimate middle-of-the-night moments with his baby, but Mom gets to have at least a few hours of uninterrupted sleep. It will definitely reduce the creeping resentment when your husband proclaims in the morning, "Wow, the baby slept all night," when you were up three times for feedings!

Pam , consultant and mother of Zach, age 18
Washington

If your hubby offers to do anything – let him, let him, let him. True, it may not get done exactly as you would like (diapering, feeding, bathing, trips to the store, etc.) but it will be one less thing for you to do. When you feel a little resentful that your husband's life hasn't seemed to be affected by the new bundle, realize that you are only jealous that you can't do what he still can (i.e., get up and read the Sunday paper — if you *can* get up, it will be to nurse the baby!). Go ahead and grieve the loss of freedom that you once had. Go ahead and get it over with so that you can willingly embrace the "bond"-age of the little life before you.

Elisabeth K. Corcoran, author of *Calm in my Chaos: Encouragement for a Mom's Weary Soul* (Kregel Publications, www.kregel.com), and mother to Sarah, age 7½, and Jack, age 6
Illinois

The husband mafia might make my husband sleep with the fishes for publicly saying this, but part of shared preparedness was planning for ways to get me some adequate sleep, since sleep-deprivation was such a huge stressor for me the first time around. How might that be accomplished, you ask? One simple rule: daddy takes the night shift the first three months. And he did. (In fact, he's still doing it and our son is nearly five months old, which maybe I shouldn't mention here since there's a chance my husband might read this and realize he could have stopped — oh, what am I saying? He's too sleep deprived to read!) Seriously, that was our deal: my husband would take care of the baby at night, getting up to change and feed him, and I would sleep and recover from bringing our son into the world. This was the best deal I ever made: my recovery time was cut in half, I was able to have the energy to deal with our other, more complicated and energetic child, and besides that, every time I'd run into someone in public they'd say, "Wow, you look great! What's your secret?" Sleep, baby; pure, uninterrupted sleep.

If you're breastfeeding, this plan is slightly more difficult to implement, since it means pumping and introducing a bottle early on, which some mothers may or may not want to do. And it's true that not every partner can be available for the night shifts, so there is a little bit of luck involved. But finding ways to get sleep—whether that means having a mom or mother-in-law stay for a few weeks, hiring a night nurse, or having someone watch your kids during the day—is a good idea. What's more, in our case the daddy night-time thing has proved to be a bonding experience not only for father and son, but for husband and wife: my husband gets it now, in a way he simply couldn't before, how exhausting and never-ending parenting is, and I get to appreciate his new-found appreciation. The first time around, I resented how he could snore through the 1, 2, 3, and 5 a.m. feedings and ask me in the morning, "How did she sleep?" This time I feel more like we're in it together.

Andrea J. Buchanan, author of *Mother Shock: Loving Every (Other) Minute of It* (Seal Press 2003), syndicated columnist, managing editor of LiteraryMama.com, and mom of two
Philadelphia

Take turns feeding the baby. I went to bed early, and my husband fed our baby at 11 pm. I would wake up for the 2 am feeding and then pump for another feeding. My husband would feed her at the 5 to 6 am feeding. Then I would feed her at the 9 am feeding and pump another bottle. This way we were getting 6 to 7 hours of sleep each.

Marie, mother of Evelyn, age 22 months
Florida

Talk with your husband throughout your pregnancy about your expectations, schedules, and needs. Identify each other's strengths and fears. Try to decide how you will share the responsibilities. My husband and I knew we wanted to share parenting as much as possible, but until the baby came we really weren't sure what that meant. Here are some things we did that helped.

1. We both wrote the thank-you cards and announcements.

2. Our son was born premature and came home after two months with lots of loud equipment that barely fit into our tiny bedroom. We decided to set up a command post in the living room and took turns sleeping on the couch and doing the middle of the night feedings. (I had pumped the whole time he was in the hospital and continued to pump extra so we had LOTS of breast milk.) We each got to get a full night's sleep every other night, and that really helped.

3. We kept a log book next to the crib to record Holden's feedings, diaper changes, etc., so that we didn't have to question what each was doing.

4. Holden had to go to the doctor quite often during the first six months home, and as much as possible, we went together or took turns taking him. That way we were able to process the information together, get to know the doctors, and not always be the "bad guy" when it came to shots.

As Holden got older we took turns every night tucking him in and every morning getting up with him. We were zealots about this because when you have a baby, even 15 minutes to yourself can be such a blessing; and knowing that you were going to have those few extra moments in bed in the morning or at night helped us make it through tough days. We still take turns tucking him in and getting him up.

We also have boy night and girl night. On Tuesdays my husband can go out and do whatever he wants — usually he plays X Box with my brother and cousin. On Wednesdays I see a movie with friends, go out to dinner, or wander through the scrapbook store. I think the time we give each other to be "us" makes us happier partners and better parents.

Connie, publisher and mother of Holden, age 3
New Jersey

Make sure your husband lets you eat, take a shower, and get fully dressed before he leaves the house after the baby is home. Otherwise, he may come home to a cranky wife who's still in her bathrobe.

Christine, lawyer and mother of Adam and Danielle
Florida

In the first three months, if you are like me, you may feel as if you are living in a soupy fog of sleep deprivation; bleary eyed from trying to attend to your precious newborn's every need. Enter Father. I had no idea that I had the best baby calming resource right under my nose. It turns out that my husband's confident, secure, and loving embrace worked like a charm. During more than one 3 am feeding, when I could not get the baby either to stop crying or nurse, he came to our rescue. Rather than feeling like chopped liver because our son wanted his father at that moment more than his mom, I was so relieved for the break and the peace that followed!

Now, lest you think it was always that simple, when the hand-off to Dad didn't work, we had to go to plan B: bouncy seat, or C: car ride, or D: a song and dance routine. It turns out that Braede loved show tunes. From birth to three months, when he awoke in the night and was seemingly inconsolable, my husband would break into his Music Man routine and sing a rousing rendition of "76 Trombones" while marching up and down our two flights of stairs, bouncing our son exuberantly in time to the music! In short order — and much to my delight— the baby was smiling and cooing. It was like magic. No matter how tired I am, seeing my husband love our son reminds me why I fell in love with him and evokes those warm, romantic feelings which help alleviate the strain a new baby can have on a marriage.

**Linda, marketing communications and mother of
Braede Bailey, age 21 months
Connecticut**

Ask for help. You are a mother, not a martyr. It took me a long time to realize that my husband could not read my mind. If I wanted his help, I needed to ask. (If he seemed content changing all the diapers and didn't ask for my help, I wouldn't offer assistance either!) Mothering is a tough job. Do not underestimate the importance of establishing – and utilizing – support. Your partner, relatives, and friends may all be glad to pitch in, but may not know you want assistance or may be reluctant to impose. Speak up and do not feel guilty. You (and your family) will be the better for it.

**Celeste Palermo, freelance writer and mother of Peyton, age 6, and Morgan, age 1
Colorado**

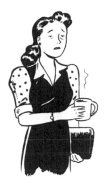

Sleeplessness

Remove the clock from your bedroom or turn it around so you can't see what time it is when you wake up to feed your newborn, and stop counting the amount of times you wake to feed. It really does make you feel better if you know you woke up during the night, not that you woke up six times for 30 to 40 minutes each time. Try and sleep with your baby if he/she wakes often. Just rolling over to feed rather than having to get up gives your body much needed rest, even if you aren't sleeping.

Lisa, La Leche League leader and mother of Keita, age 10, Sharra, age 7½, and Siabhaon, age 5

Keep your sense of perspective. If your sleeping situation isn't working for you and you're too tired to function, feel free to change it, but do it gently. There had been many times when, as I sat in my rocker for what seemed like hours trying to get my babies to sleep, I remembered how many would-be mothers – some struggling with infertility issues or parents with severely ill children – would have loved to be in my shoes – holding, rocking, and nursing their own babies. With my second child this was easier because I could remember being in the same situation with my firstborn, and I know now how short a time those "problems" last. My four year old, who was never forced to "sleep through the night," now sleeps so soundly that he could fall out of bed and still be snoozing!

Hannah, mother of Ian, age 4, and Eliza, age 13 months
South Carolina

Nighttime sleep is the most valuable sleep in helping you recover. Five hours of uninterrupted sleep per night is required for brain restoration because it gives you a full sleep cycle. The baby can be fed with breast milk or formula in the bottle. You need to be "off duty" physically, emotionally, and psychologically. You can either split the night with your partner or alternate taking a full night "on," then a full night "off," If your partner is not home, you will need to enlist a support person to be responsible for the baby during this time. When you are "off" you should sleep away from the baby in another room, with earplugs. Many of our clients also use a fan, air purifier, or another appliance to block all baby noises. When your partner is "off," he can use the same techniques.

Remember, it is your job to take care of yourself. Even if you cannot arrange for this nightly, a few nights a week will help. If you are able to nap in the day, do so, but it does not replace nighttime sleep. Sleep problems occur frequently with mood disorders. If you are unable to sleep at night when everyone else is sleeping, please talk to your health practitioner. Medication will be helpful.

Shoshana S. Bennett, Ph.D., mother of Elana and Aaron and Pec Indman, Ed.D., MFT, mother of Megan and Emily: co-authors of *Beyond the Blues, A Guide to Understanding and Treating Prenatal and Postpartum Depression*
California

Rest when the baby rests. Don't clean house, etc. Those early morning feedings are killers. Parents need rest, too, and they shouldn't be afraid to nap or limit their activities/involvements while baby is little.

Sue, RN, LCCE , and mother of Angie, age 20
Minnesota

When you're up for the second, third, or gazillionth time during the night to feed or soothe your newborn and you feel it's never going to end…use your head! What I mean by that is talk to yourself positively, saying things like: "This too shall pass," "This won't last forever," "Other moms are doing this right now," "I can do it," and "My baby needs me." And remember, just because you're saying these things doesn't mean you can't cry. Cry, feed, and help yourself stay positive.

Nicole, doula and mother of Alanna, age 8, Braden, age 6, Danielle, age 3, and Ethan, age 2 months
Canada

I have heard so often of overly tired parents. I (amazingly) found myself getting more sleep after my baby was born than when I was pregnant. Why? Because every time I could get her down for a decent nap, I made myself sleep as well. It really diffused the stress I felt from waking every two hours to feed her at night. Yes, some dishes went undone, and some laundry awaited me when I woke. But an infant is incredibly portable and adjustable, and I found I could actually do these things while she was awake. Even if the house was a mess at the end of the day, I had infinitely more patience for my daughter and was able to be cheerful for my husband, because I had managed to cobble together eight hours of sleep throughout the night and day. Don't feel guilty and get some rest. I slept with my little one in the same bed, but even if that is not for you, put him/her in the bassinet or crib, lie down, and get some sleep. Sleep is such an important rejuvenator, and you will have much more joy if you allow yourself the rest that you need and deserve!

Renee, Web designer and stay-at-home mother of Alexandria, age 2
California

I've yet to hear a parent tell me that she or he loves getting up throughout the night to tend to a baby's needs. As much as we adore our little bundles, it's tough when you're woken up over and over again, night after night. Since it's a fact that your baby will be waking you up, you may as well make yourself as comfortable as possible. The first step is to learn to relax about night wakings right now. Being stressed or frustrated about having to get up won't change a thing. The situation will improve day by day; and before you know it, your little newborn won't be so little anymore — she'll be walking and talking and getting into everything in sight…during the day, and sleeping peacefully all night long.

Elizabeth Pantley, author of *The No-Cry Sleep Solution: Gentle Ways to Help Your Baby Sleep Through the Night* (Excerpted with permission by McGraw-Hill/ Contemporary Publishing. www.pantley.com/elizabeth) and mother of Angela, age 17, Vanessa, age 15, David, age 14, and Coleton, age 5
Washington

Enjoy those quiet moments in the middle of the night when it is just the two of you – even if it is 3 am. They are over far too quickly.

Kara, mother of Kyle, age 11 months
New Jersey

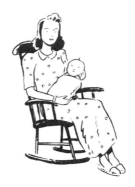

— Adjusting to a New Life —

During the first year (and I suspect much, much longer), be okay
with winging it. Every once in a while I try to step back and say,
"There are far stupider and lazier parents out there, and their kids
are turning out (or have turned out) just fine...thriving even!" I am
so not a good schedule person. And early on when I was trying to
get William on a schedule, I thought – how the hell can I do that
when I don't have a schedule. It turns out that we kind of have one
anyway – so I guess this all boils down to "relax and go with it."

Alicia, mother of William, age 1
New Jersey

Stop waiting for life to return to "normal." Life as you knew it, will
never be "normal" again. This is a time to redefine what is "normal."
It's a time to be extra gentle with your expectations of yourself
while you readjust to your new life with baby.

Sarah Zeldman, Life Balance coach – Balanced Woman Coaching,
www.Balanced-woman-coaching.com,
and mother of Yosef, age 3½, and Shanya, age 1
New York

There will be good days and bad days. Dwell on the good ones.

Jennifer, recruiter and mother of Blake and Madeline, age 2½ years
Pennsylvania

"This too shall pass"…a phrase that has kept me strong, kept me sane, and allowed me to look at hard times with a smile, knowing everything will be okay. We need to embrace the precious years of our children, giving them our all with a positive outlook. I sure have grown as a mother knowing "this too shall pass."

Jennifer, mother of Cameron, age 3½, and Makenzie, age 2
New Jersey

Learn to laugh at messes because there will be plenty of them.

Beckie, mother of Alyssa, 10 months
Texas

You will not clean the house every day. You will not clean yourself every day. You will not get everything done that you plan to get done every day. You'll just be in the moment, aiming to meet the small goals of fed kids and clean hands, and little by little you'll make it work.

The more you fight this idea of surrendering to smaller, more manageable goals, the harder life is. So surrender. And remember: nothing lasts longer than three months, not the good stages ("Hey, she's sleeping through the night!"), not the bad stages ("Oh, my God, this kid wakes up every hour on the hour!").

Of course, it's different for everyone. But for me, letting go of the idea that everything around me has to be perfect in order for me to feel perfect has been crucial. I have a chaotic life now, but that doesn't mean that I'm a mess. The pre-kid me would probably be saying, "Yes, you are!" But now, after figuring it out the hard way, I know better.

Andrea J. Buchanan, author of *Mother Shock: Loving Every (Other) Minute of It* (Seal Press 2003), syndicated columnist, managing editor of LiteraryMama.com, and mother of two
Philadelphia

Realize babies make messes and enjoy the toys everywhere.

Michele, doula, massage therapist, and mother of Jacob, age 9, Skylar, age 5, and Autumn, age 15 months
New Jersey

You can still have it all, just not all at once.

Sandy, physical therapist and mother of Marika, age 4, and Haley, age 1
California

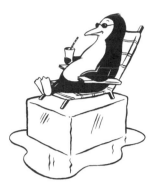

Keeping Your Cool

As a childbirth educator and OB/RN, I asked a social worker one time what I could do to prevent child abuse. She suggested time-outs for parents. I tell my parents that even though they love their baby, there will be times when they don't enjoy being parents. Perhaps the baby won't quit crying or has kept them up all night, and they are exhausted, etc. It is then I suggest they put the baby in his/her room and take a short 10 to 15 minute time-out. Perhaps take a relaxing shower, turn up the music and sing loudly, exercise, deep breathe, or call someone to vent to, or better yet, to come relieve you so you can get out of the house for a while. I tell them it is not what you think about doing but what you do. I reassure them that they are good parents even if they have moments when they don't like or can't handle the job. I also teach them why babies cry and what to do to comfort them, plus encourage parents to take time for themselves each day, if only to go for a short walk and think about something other than baby. Babies are wonderful but very demanding.

Sue, RN, LCCE, and mother of Angie, age 20
Minnesota

Always practice patience and stay calm when your child is worked up. As hard as that may be, you will see that your child will quickly calm down too once he sees that you are not out of control. There is no need to spank, yell, or get upset. Always remain calm and reasonable – children learn what they see.

Anonymous

If your baby picks up on your stress, he/she will behave appropriately!

**Tamalyn Roberts, Web site owner, www.names2be.com, and mother of
Natalie, age 9, Matthew, age 7, and Paul, age 5
Anglesey, United Kingdom**

When your kids are cranky and the dog has just peed on the floor; the phone is ringing but you can't find it because it's lost in the recliner chair; the mailman came but all he brought was junk; and you haven't had a square meal, and you're waiting for reinforcements to arrive – gather the children (and the dog, if you like), put on a CD of music YOU like, and DANCE. After your children stare at you for awhile, they will soon want to be like you and DANCE the day away, too.

**Courtney Crow Wyrtzen, certified birth doula and mother of Blythe, age 2½ Hip Hop
You Don't Stop Rockin Dancer, and Fiona, age 1 Ballerina Gliding Butterfly
Texas**

In those wee hours of the morning – when I was so tired I could cry; and I was up with my little son for the fourth or fifth or tenth time of the night, nursing him to sleep; and I was so angry and resentful – I had a little trick to turn it all around and prevent the angry thoughts from pervading my mind and tainting my attitude toward him. I just tried as hard as I could to think of one thing he had done that day to make me smile. There was always something, and I always managed to conjure it up. Just thinking of his little face and the little person who needed me, rather than this duty I had, made it all better for another hour or so until he woke up again.

**Jessica Hudson, owner of Eva Lillian maternity, www.evalillian.com, and mother of
Julian, age 3, and Eva, age 1
Michigan**

The children who are the hardest to love are the ones that need it the most.

**Barbara, service specialist and mother of William, age 34, and Robert, age 30
New Jersey**

When your children melt down in the grocery store, when they use your house plants as sandboxes, when they throw the homemade baby food at your with vigor…breathe, and nothing else. You can correct them in a nanosecond; but at that moment, oxygen is all you need.

**Wendy, counselor and mother of Katie, age 14 months, and second on the way
New Jersey**

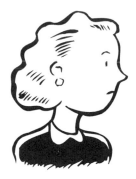

—Postpartum Depression—

Be sure your partner, family, and close friends learn the signs of postpartum depression before you give birth. Having suffered from PPD for about a year after the birth of my first child, I know the depressed new mom will probably not be willing or able to contact her doctor or midwife and say, "I think I'm depressed, and I need help" on her own. It would have been so helpful if my family members had recognized my depression and encouraged me to get the professional help I needed.

Patti Newton, childbirth educator, doula, freelance writer, and mother of Jordan, age 13, Becky, age 8, and Annie, age 7
New Jersey

We encourage you to contact Postpartum Support International (PSI) at (805) 967-7636 or www.postpartum.net to locate a therapist who has shown interest and commitment in the postpartum field. PSI, along with other organizations in the Resources section, provides specialized training in perinatal mood disorders. We have not found any graduate training that covers this material. Do not assume (as many insurance companies would like you to believe) that someone who has expertise in working with depression or other mood disorders is knowledgeable about perinatal mood disorders.

Shoshana S. Bennett, Ph.D., mother of Elana and Aaron and Pec Indman, Ed.D., MFT, mother of Megan and Emily: co-authors of *Beyond the Blues, A Guide to Understanding and Treating Prenatal and Postpartum Depression*
California

I suffered severe postpartum depression after my first baby. Interestingly, despite everything we now know about this disease, it took several middle-of-the-night phone calls and trips to the emergency room before the doctors believed me that I was depressed. Trust your instincts. If you find yourself thinking, "I just don't feel right," don't ignore your feelings. If your doctor dismisses you with, "Ah, you'll get over it," find a new doctor! You are not alone and there IS help.

Sarah Smiley, syndicated columnist and mother of Ford, age 4, and Owen, age 2
Florida

While I had heard of the "Baby Blues" and had read up on the subject of what to expect after the birth of my baby, I was surprised by the magnitude of emotions I felt for a few weeks following my son's arrival. I knew it was hormonal and normal, but the emotions – the crying, fear, uncertainty – coupled with exhaustion and learning to breastfeed affected my mood greatly. I had imagined feeling blissful; and while I was indeed very happy, I couldn't stop crying. Fortunately for me, the feelings began to subside by my 6-week postpartum checkup. I knew that I did not have PPD, though what I had experienced was indeed the "Baby Blues." It's important for new moms to know that if these feelings occur, it's a part of the process.

Get support through a partner, spouse, or friend, and talk to your doctor if symptoms don't go away. Being a new mother is an awe-inspiring, amazing feeling, but it can be a difficult adjustment for some.

Being aware that this normal hormonal "letdown" may occur is important so you know how to take care of your heart and soul as well as your mind during those first few weeks following the birth.

Jo Gerard, consultant, writer, and mother of a baby boy, age 8 months
Wisconsin

When we're depressed or anxious, the four walls feel as if they're closing in. Our world feels darker and smaller. We tend to fold in emotionally and physically (as in crossing our arms, hunching over, and fixing our gaze downward). To counter this, go outside your home, look up at the sky, stand up straight, put your arms at your sides, and breathe. You don't have to actually go anywhere. Just go outside once a day, even if this means standing outside your front door in your bathrobe.

Shoshana S. Bennett, Ph.D., mother of Elana and Aaron and Pec Indman, Ed.D., MFT, mother of Megan and Emily: co-authors of *Beyond the Blues, A Guide to Understanding and Treating Prenatal and Postpartum Depression*
California

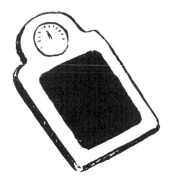

— Your Postpartum Body —

Use cabbage leaves for engorged breasts: they really work. I found that kind of scrunching them up (to release the juice in the veins), then unfolding them and putting them vein-side touching the breast right in the bra helps alleviate pain.

Jill, accountant/HR and mother of Sara, age 8, and Ethan, age 1
Canada

Several weeks after you have a C-section and you can touch your belly comfortably, place both your hands, finger tips only, on your incision. Move the skin first up then down and side to side several times a day. This will make the tissues that have grown together and become hard nice and soft. It will get to the point where you will have to actually look for your scar; you will no longer feel it.

Dawn, birth doula and mother of
Stephanie, age 19, Peter, age 17, Craig, age 10, and Kimberly, age 8
Maryland

Don't freak out when your hair starts falling out about three months postpartum. It's a totally normal process that your hair follicles go through, as they did not shed themselves normally during the pregnancy and are making up for lost time!

Diana, professional clarinet player and mother of
Anna, age 2, and newborn Simon
New York

Pregnant mothers will be encouraged to nurse their babies and told that one of the side effects is that it burns calories, and your pregnancy weight will "just fall off." It's a lie!!! Definitely nurse your babies because it's great for them, but don't check the scale afterwards.

Anonymous

As soon as you feel able, go out and buy yourself a pair of jeans or jean shorts that fit your newly nonpregnant body. Don't worry about the size. You will feel great being in nonmaternity, nonstretchy clothes, and your mom friends will be amazed that you are back in "your" jeans already. Just smile and say, "Thank you."

Robin, LPN, and mother of Ian, age 9, Colin, age 6, and Shannon, age 9 months
Arizona

The uterus is actually the only floating organ in your body. It is suspended by two ligaments. If you try to be a supermom and run errands, clean the house, and so on without giving those ligaments time to heal, you will regret it later. Many women feel well enough to go to the mall with their two-day-old baby, but this is terribly unwise. Acquire help and stay in bed with your baby as much as possible. Only rest in a reclined position will truly allow those ligaments to heal properly. The results of not allowing proper healing include a possible prolapsed uterus later down the road. You aren't being lazy while resting with your baby. Newlyweds get a honeymoon. (It is called that because it used to last a whole month.) You may not be able to spare a whole month of letting others pamper you, but try to take as long of a "babymoon" as you can. It's good for your baby, and it's good for you!

Sharon, midwife in training and mother of Zachary, age 12, Alex, age 10, Timothy, age 8, Juliann, age 4, Daniel, age 2 in heaven, and Matthew, age 1
Kansas

I was weak from being on bed rest for 20 weeks and was surprised at the soreness in my upper back from holding a 9-pound baby. If you can, hold a couple of hand weights and do some lat pull-downs in the month before delivery. If you have been working out your whole pregnancy, this might not be a problem for you. Also, I was surprised that I was constantly sweating for the month after birth. You know all that water you are carrying? It has to leave somehow.

The contributing moms of "The List," a growing list
of new mom tips passed from friend to friend
New Jersey, Maryland, and Delaware

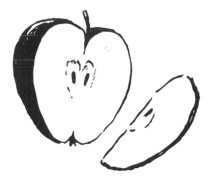

Your Health

Remember to put yourself first on your list of things to take care of after you come home with your baby. Taking good care of yourself is not a luxury, as many think: it is essential. Sometimes, it seems too simple to be true, but your baby needs you to eat well, sleep well, rest as much as possible, and get out in the sunshine and fresh air. Avoid things and people that make you feel bad. Surround yourself with giggles and hugs. Take a walk, a warm bath, or a slow deep breath whenever you can. Do not expect too much from yourself. Do not push yourself too hard. Say "yes" when others offer to help and tell them what they can do for you. Remind yourself that things aren't always going to go the way you want them to. Screen phone calls. Expect and accept any negative feelings. Avoid overdoing anything. Be careful not to ask too many people for advice. Prioritize what needs to be done and what can wait. Above all, rest when your baby sleeps – the thank-you notes can wait!

Karen Kleiman, MSW, clinical director of The Postpartum Stress Center,
www.postpartumstress.com
Pennsylvania

Remember that one of the important things you do to take care of your child is to take care of yourself!

Lisa, art therapist and mother of
Joshua, Ariel, Atara, Emmuna, Daniella, and Elyakim
Lower Galilee, Israel

Being a mom is the best job in the world, but in order to be the best mom in the world we need to take care of ourselves. I personally went through a very scary experience by not taking care of myself. Once I learned that by having my own goals and dreams I became a better mom, my entire family benefited.

Tracy Lyn Moland, author of *Mom Management, Managing Mom Before Everybody Else* and mother of Courtney-Lyn, age 8, and Mats, age 6
Canada

My advice is more a concept. The beauty of motherhood is the self-sacrifice — the strange and unnatural notion NOT to do what is best for yourself, but for your children. The maternal overpowers even the most selfish of us. The self-sacrifice has a duality, the light and the dark. For the light, throughout the day I remind myself of a certain saying. I have it on my refrigerator. "1. I am Lucky. 2. I am Blessed. 3. Enjoy them. 4. They grow up too fast." On the darker side of the self-sacrifice moon is the thought — "Take care of yourself first, then you can take care of others. If you're hungry or frazzled or exhausted, you can not be a good mom." Reminding your children of your needs on occasion is no bad thing.

This morning's events inspired me with the above. The Hounds, Shae and Keira, had eaten breakfast. I had not eaten, had hunger. I helped Shae get settled into an activity— "Mom get me a pencil. Get me paper. Get me glue." Keira was also a constant source of needs. The list was growing. I had to stop the "to do" list and state that I really had to eat breakfast. Big eyes looked back at me as if to say, "Oh you're human like me?" Of course, while eating my buttered toast and eggs, I shared and gave up the last best bite for Keira.
Motherhood.

Jane, mother of Shae, age 5, and Keira, age 2
Pennsylvania

Bodywork – massage, shiatsu, craniosacral therapy, chiropractic, acupuncture, and more – is great for bodily comfort and ease of movement, yet also for peace of mind. Find someone to help you through this big change! Women become emotionally stronger when well cared for, so the baby is therefore also feeling better!

Diane Hynes, shiatsu/craniosacral practitioner and mother of Taegan, age 28 months
New Jersey

Often women with postpartum depression and anxiety crave sweets and carbohydrates. If you can eat something nutritious, especially protein, each time you feed the baby, you can help keep your blood sugar level even. This will contribute to keeping your mood stable. We understand this may be difficult if you are experiencing a lack of appetite, so do the best you can. If you have trouble eating, try drinking your food – for example, protein shakes or drinks. Avoid caffeine.

Ask a support person to stock your refrigerator with things like yogurt, sliced deli meat and cheese, hardboiled eggs, precut vegetables, and fruit. Better yet, if they are not already offering, ask people to bring you food. Don't forget to drink water – dehydration can increase anxiety. Appetite problems are quite common with postpartum depression and anxiety. Please tell your health practitioner about any appetite changes. It might be helpful to consult a nutritionist who is familiar with depression and anxiety when you have the energy.

Shoshana S. Bennett, Ph.D., mother of Elana and Aaron and Pec Indman, Ed.D., MFT, mother of Megan and Emily: co-authors of *Beyond the Blues, A Guide to Understanding and Treating Prenatal and Postpartum Depression* California

Make sure you're setting a good example while eating and providing meals and snacks. Parents and children should pretty much be eating the same things. If you are "on a diet" that isn't fit for your child, then it is not fit for you. If you're giving your children food that you wouldn't eat because it would "make you fat," then it's not good for your kids either! Nutritious, whole food eating is good for every age group. Start good eating habits right away by eating good foods for yourself and then breastfeed your baby. Babies will enjoy the foods their moms eat by getting accustomed to the taste of breast milk.

Watching Mom snack on carrot sticks and apples will make Junior want a bit of apple, too. If Mom is following some crazy fad in the name of "diet" or "losing weight," the kids will file that away for later. Plus, if you wouldn't consider the diet healthy for kids, then it's not healthy for you either!

Stacy Walker, wellness encourager, www.Manna4Me.com, and mother of Shayne, age 8, Harris Anne, age 6, David, age 4, and Hudson, age 1 Alabama

Find a way to steal 30 minutes a day for yourself. A sane mommy makes a happy child.

Robbie, mother of Holl, age 2 Texas

The rapid decline in the levels of the hormones estrogen and progesterone after birth can lead to the notorious "Baby Blues." This depression of spirits is common and quite normal, but nonetheless disturbing. It varies from one woman to another in how severe this depression might be and how long it will last. It is usually something that lifts after a few days, and some women do not suffer with it at all. The Bach Remedies, although very gentle, can be of great help; and if taken straight away, before the depression has had a chance to dig its heels in, so much the better. Everyone has their own individual personalities and characteristics; and so it follows that we should treat ourselves in an individual way, choosing the remedies as to who we are, how we are, and why we feel the way we do. The following are a few suggestions of remedies that might be helpful:

* The reason for the baby blues is unknown: The mother is overjoyed to have a baby, has a loving partner and a secure home, but a cloud of gloom overshadows it. For these women it can be difficult to fathom as there is no account for this feeling: Mustard

* The reason for the baby blues is known: The mother has had stitches, and they are really uncomfortable; or the baby is not behaving how you would expect him/her to. The mother feels disappointed or disheartened for a known reason: Gentian

* The mother not coping very well and has a fear of loosing control: Cherry Plum, Rescue Remedy

* Women who are constantly expecting more from themselves or feeling guilty for not doing enough: Pine

* Those who are not grounded; are in a dream world and not really aware of what is happening around them; are feeling detached from reality: Clematis

* Women having difficulty adjusting to having a baby: Walnut

* Women who are bravely coping but not caring for themselves: Oak

* Women who are overanxious and fearful about the baby's well-being: Red Chestnut

* Women who have suffered a traumatic birth: Star of Bethlehem, Rescue Remedy

**Bettina Rasmussen, co-owner of PlatyPaws Soft Soles Baby Shoes
and mother of Dylan, age 3
California**

Do whatever you have to do to survive: sleep together; let them watch TV to get them to eat; sleep in late if the baby is sleeping.

**Anita, playcenter owner and mother of
Nicholas, age 3, Olivia, age 2, and Sam, age 5 months
Florida**

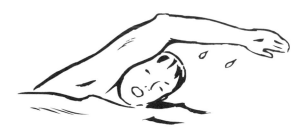

— Exercise After Baby —

Include your baby in your postpartum exercise routine instead of trying to squeeze in exercise between naps and feedings. You will retone your body more quickly, and you'll be teaching your baby the benefits of physical activity right from the beginning.

**Lisa Stone, pre/postnatal fitness specialist and mother of
Emma, age 15½, Savannah, age 13, and Morgan, age 8
Georgia**

I didn't want to leave my baby to exercise, so I brought her along to StrollerFit – Exercise With Your Baby Class! I was able to spend time with her, watch her interact, as well as make some friends of my own and get an incredible workout in 50 minutes!

**Kelly Rodgers, fitness specialist and mother of Isabella, age 10 months
Texas**

Take time for your health and fitness. Allowing yourself to get back in shape is great, but the real perk is the one you will get after a great workout. Taking the time to be fit and healthy can give a lift to a not so great day of motherhood.

**Jennifer Lungren, fitness instructor for Stroller Strides™ and mother of
a daughter, age 20 months
Virginia**

Exercising during the time period that you are breastfeeding can present some interesting dilemmas. As a pretty small-chested woman before pregnancy I was astonished at the changes in my body during and after pregnancy. To alleviate some of the bounce and pain present during the months that I was breastfeeding, I found that two sports bras worn at the same time was the answer. This is in reference to medium/high impact activities. This change in my wardrobe made all the difference in my enjoyment during exercise.

Laurie Bagley, owner of Fit Maternity & Beyond and mother of Avriel, age 7

If you want to buy exercise videos to get back into shape, make sure they are the kind that you can do WITH your baby. That way, you'll have one less thing to do while the baby naps.

Sarah Zeldman, Life Balance coach – Balanced Woman Coaching,
www. Balanced-woman-coaching.com,
and mother of Yosef, age 3½, and Shanya, age 1
New York

As soon as you feel up to it, put your baby in a front carrier and go hiking! The fresh air will do you both wonders and will kindle your spirit for the outdoors – something every child's mother should have!

Joy, owner of Colorado Mountain Mamas and mother of Amanda, age 2
Colorado

Transitioning into pregnancy and early motherhood is the first of many letting goes. It means letting go of your old physical and emotional self, your pre-pregnancy body, and pre-motherhood ideas of what should get done, how it should be done, and how expeditiously it should get done. It can take some time to get comfortable with this new person who you are growing into. When learning to let go and make the transition, have patience with yourself. You have the rest of your life to figure it out. On the journey, remember that no one actually lives at the center of the universe, but that we all need to be nurtured. Realize and honor your needs by making them known. Find solace in numbers by joining a prenatal or postpartum yoga program where you can be supported during the ride.

Gail Silver, owner of Yoga Child and mother of Ben, age 5, and Anabel, age 3
Pennsylvania

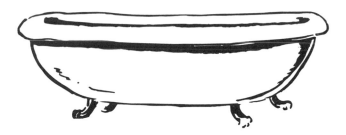

Time for Yourself

Of course you can enjoy a hot shower! Place baby in a bouncer seat in the bathroom while you shower. If you don't have glass shower doors, simply purchase a clear vinyl shower curtain, and entertain baby with funny faces while delighting in some time for Mom! As baby gets older, add a laundry basket of toys to play with instead of the bouncer seat.

**Sheryl Fernandez, owner of Bellies and Bubbles Maternity
and mother of Dalton, age 16 months
Pennsylvania**

If you go out for an evening, try not to feel guilty about leaving your baby in capable hands so you can enjoy yourself. It is important for your mental health to treat yourself to some time away from being a mom.

**Wendy, March of Dimes employee and mother to Brier, age 4
Wisconsin**

Running your home is truly a lot like running a business. Bring some of your time management and work skills home with you so that you have more time to enjoy being a mom.

**Tracy Lyn Moland, author of
Mom Management, Managing Mom Before Everybody Else
and mother of Courtney-Lyn, age 8, and Mats, age 6
Canada**

Remember to take your shower first in the morning and get ready before the baby. If your baby is not sleeping, let he or she lie in a rocker baby seat and place it right by the shower where he/she can see you. The visual appearance of you and the sound of the shower is relaxing. Remember, you are important, too!

**Jamie Yasko-Mangum, certified image consultant and mother of
Stone, age 4½, and Spencer, age 2½
Florida**

I always took time first thing in the AM before the babies woke up. I always took at least one class for myself. I went grocery shopping at midnight: I shopped in bulk, and I shopped once a month except for dairy and bread. I froze milk and allowed it to thaw at room temperature.

**Melanie, full-time domestic engineer, educator, author, and mother of twins
Meldonár and Meldoníque
Massachusetts**

The myth is that if we really love our children enough, we don't need breaks from them. This certainly isn't the case! We've bought into the idea that taking time for ourselves is selfish and bad, and therefore we feel guilty when we even think we need a break. The truth is that all good mothers take breaks – that's how they stay good mothers! We strongly recommend that you get regularly scheduled time off at least three times a week for a minimum of two hours at a time. For every job other than being a mother, breaks are mandated by law, and you'd expect much more time off.

**Shoshana S. Bennett, Ph.D., mother of Elana and Aaron and Pec Indman, Ed.D., MFT,
mother of Megan and Emily: co-authors of *Beyond the Blues, A Guide to
Understanding and Treating Prenatal and Postpartum Depression*
California**

Even though it is hard, never, ever forget yourself. Even if you feel totally selfish, make sure you take time for yourself. It teaches your child that each person is special enough to have his/her wants and needs met…a hard lesson to learn unless you grown up seeing it taught by example.

**Abby, mother of Joey, age 7, Alyssa, age 5, Nicholas, age 3, and Seth,
age 10 months
Kansas**

I believe there is a guilt switch in our brain that turns on as soon as we give birth! Even though we often know better, as moms we feel guilty for so many things. We feel guilty for feeling guilty. As a mom we need to learn that self care, saying no, and delegation make us better moms. Just because we need some time alone or have a hobby does not make us a bad mom. Why, I believe it makes us a much better mom. When we say no to someone else's request, we are also saying yes to ourselves or our family. When we delegate, we are providing our children with powerful tools to help them become responsible adults. So moms, right now turn off the guilt switch in your brain!

Tracy Lyn Moland, author of
Mom Management, Managing Mom Before Everybody Else
and mother of Courtney-Lyn, age 8, and Mats, age 6
Canada

If there is something you have always wanted to do – some dream, goal, or passion – then start to take some steps toward it. Don't put it on hold because you're a mother. It isn't selfish to make time for yourself – it's selfish NOT to! Once you are a mother, you are your children's role model, so it's even more important to live your best life. If you don't, you're not just cheating yourself, you're cheating your kids, too. Madonna said that motherhood was inspiring for her because "I wanted to understand what I was going to teach my daughter. I didn't really understand where I stood on things. I think that was my wake-up call. I wanted to understand how I was going to go about finding true and lasting happiness in my life and how I was going to teach that to my daughter." After I had my first daughter, I started to pursue my dream of doing stand-up comedy. I started with a 3-hour class once a week for 10 weeks. The class gave me such a boost of energy. For three hours each week, I wasn't a mom, wife, daughter, or friend. I was just ME! That's the person I want my daughter to know in her life.

Sally Robertson, life coach and mother of Eva, age 5, and Francesca, age 3
New Jersey

Love your child, enjoy the bonding, meet the needs of this little being, and remember that by respecting and honoring YOURSELF, you teach your child self care. If you are hurting, sick, angry, or uncomfortable, saying NO to your child will teach your child to honor his/her body and feelings and say NO when he/she needs to.

Dori, healer and mother of Kyler, age 2
New Jersey

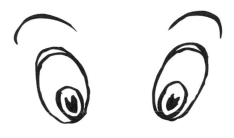

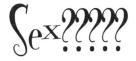

In case your close friends with kids have not mentioned it, sex after delivery can be downright painful! You can blame your out-of-whack hormones. Even after waiting the required 6 weeks for your doctor's approval, regaining intimacy may be a slow process with lots of moans and groans (not the good kind!). It does get better again, so don't lose hope, but it may take months. I advise you to stock up on lots of lubricant to ease the transition!

Kate, advertising account supervisor and mother of Jackson, age 4 months
Pennsylvania

When my son was born, I delivered with a midwife on a birthing stool, and he swooshed out in one solid push before I had any idea what was happening. Because of gravity and the force of my push, I had a second degree tear to my perineum as well as a tiny tear in the front. The midwife stitched, and four months later, the scar tissue made me feel as though I was still trussed up like a Thanksgiving turkey. I looked to online parenting communities for advice and support and was told that with time, things would go back to normal. Sex continued to be uncomfortable probably until 10 months after giving birth; but, sure enough, we found that with time and patience, careful maneuvering, and stock in AstroGlide, things were fine.

Kathleen, mother of Alejandro, age almost 3, and
twins Nieves and Paloma, age 9 months
New Jersey

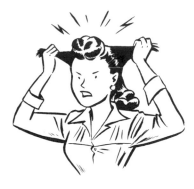

— Breastfeeding Blues —

Breastfeeding isn't always as easy as the experts make it sound. The first 6 to 8 weeks are really hard. It's important to get support and guidance during this time. It is very easy to give up, especially if it is not going smoothly. The hospital does not always do a great job with giving breastfeeding moms the kind of support they need.

Kerry, psychotherapist and mother of Benjamin, age 6 months
Maryland

Don't feel like you are not a good mother if you don't like breast-feeding. Many of my friends and I talked about our experiences breastfeeding and agreed that it's not as easy as we had thought it would be. It's draining (no pun intended), physically and emotional-ly, and it doesn't just happen perfectly by instinct. I had so much trouble with my son Lou, but I suffered though it because I thought I had to. Then with my daughter Emmy, I had trouble again, and my lactation consultant even told me (after several tearful visits) that it should be a good experience; and if I was going back to work in the next few months, I should just bottle feed and enjoy my time with my new daughter. I cannot tell you how much more relaxed I have been with her since I stopped. No doubt, breastfeeding is so good for the baby and can be a wonderful bonding experience between a mother and child; but if you have trouble, seek help and don't feel badly if you decide to stop sooner than you had hoped.

Tara, high school teacher and mother of Lou, age 2½, and Emmy, age 10 weeks
Tennessee

Many mothers become frustrated with breastfeeding because they are unable to quantify the amount of milk an infant drinks. Please remember that breast milk is chock full of healthy proteins that formulas are unable to replicate. Your baby will benefit from breast milk physically (studies show less obesity in breastfed children), emotionally (an irreversible bond with Mommy), and intellectually (studies have shown children who are breastfed have higher IQ's). Do not get discouraged if baby does not follow a "prescribed" feeding schedule. All babies are different and will eat only what they require. As long as baby is pooping, peeing, and growing, he/she is getting what is needed for a great start at life.

Dr. Amy Callaghan, physician and mother of Natalie, age 5, and Sean, age 3½
South Dakota

I had a difficult time with painful nursing. I was so ready to give up, but I just toughed it out. After eight weeks it all changed. The pain was gone, and I had a wonderful relationship nursing with my son. So many people do not have the support they need. Seek and find a support group on the internet or a person in town and stick it out. Nursing is the most rewarding experience you will ever have.

Kimberly, stay-at-home mother of
Haiden, age 9, Karsyn, age 5, and Nathan, age 6 months
Alabama

Build your network of breastfeeding support people during your pregnancy. Your list should include professionals, such as breastfeeding educators, lactation consultants, and midwives, as well as moms who have successfully breastfed their babies. Being able to reach for your support list on your most difficult days of breastfeeding will make it easier for you to work through your difficulties and continue breastfeeding. Many women fail to seek support and quickly stop breastfeeding, saying they couldn't produce enough milk or their baby wasn't "getting enough." How successful you are with breastfeeding depends on how determined you are to breastfeed your baby. Most difficulties can be worked through, but you have to reach out and ask for help when you need it.

Patti Newton, childbirth educator, doula, freelance writer, and mother of
Jordan, age 13, Becky, age 8, Annie, age 7
New Jersey

This is definitely an art and takes a lot of time and perseverance to get it right. It certainly didn't come naturally to me.

Michelle, office manager and mother of Brooklyn, age 18 months

When we found out I was pregnant, I decided that I would breastfeed my baby. I thought that this is a natural thing that all mothers do, so how hard could it be. Breastfeeding is hard but don't give up – everyone finds their own rhythm. Do your best and you and your child will be happier than you can imagine.

Alicynn, mother of Grace, age 18 months
Massachusetts

Breastfeeding is the most rewarding and enjoyable part of raising a baby. If you stick with it for the first few weeks, it gets easier, more rewarding, and more enjoyable.

Wendy, stay-at-home mother of Tyler, age 8, and Alyssa, age 1
Colorado

Plan to breastfeed. Don't say "I'm going to try to breastfeed." For thousands of years, this was the only way to feed babies.Clearly, it is something you can and should do. Find a friend who has breastfed or call your local La Leche League leader and line up your support for success.

Stephanie, mother of Kate, age 8, and Ben, age 6
Maryland

As soon as a sore spot from a plugged duct is noticed in the breast, position baby so that the baby's chin is pointing towards the spot and nurse. This may require some help. There were many nights in the first few weeks when my husband would hold my newborn upside down to nurse from a position that would help ease the pain.

Marisa, mother of Elijah, age 2½, and Marin, age 9 months
California

If you are having a hard time breastfeeding in those early days after leaving the hospital, call a lactation consultant for a home visit. Generally, in less than an hour she can identify what's causing you pain and frustration and have you nursing comfortably. They do charge a fee, but it's only a small fraction of what you'd spend on formula, not to mention the stress that goes away when you learn to nurse like a pro in your own home.

Shelly Drouin, StrollerFit instructor and mother of Haley, age 21 months
Texas

The "trick" to lactation is that there was no trick to lactation! There is no one right answer. Everyone had to find out what is right for them, their body, and their baby. My sisters had no problems. They didn't even own a breast pump. I had lots of problems, but eventually met with success. Other friends of mine had so many problems that they couldn't continue. While I think no one would argue that breast milk is the healthiest and most natural choice for an infant, the adage "breast is best" can put undue pressure on women. What's best should be what's best for you and your baby. Women shouldn't be afraid to ask for help. (I found a wonderful nurse/consultant from the La Leche Web site after Anne came home.) But for some people breastfeeding just doesn't work out for them, even though they try. Breastfeeding my daughter was one of the most wonderful experiences for me. I felt I gave her a gift to help her grow stronger while she was in the hospital. It was a beautiful bonding experience. But it wasn't easy, and it certainly wasn't what I was expecting. Fortunately, we were able to make it work.

Dr. Beth, developmental psychologist and educator and mother of Anne, age 1, and Jack, age 1 month
Massachusetts

Don't be fooled into thinking that prior knowledge (from books, classes, or other children) means you will have the expected results. Until you have DONE it with THAT baby, you can't really predict whether your baby will latch right away or not. If not, remember it's a learning curve for both you and baby. Get any help that's out there: ask the hospital, lactation consultant, or your local La Leche League leader. There are many, many people out there who want to help you succeed. Stick with it, make small goals for yourself, and promise yourself you won't give up without professional help. You CAN do it!

Beth Foster, certified lactation consultant, consultant for Natural Family Boutique, and mother of Nicholas, age 5, Alexander, age 3, and Baby #3 due in March '05.
Kentucky

La Leche League's mother to mother support was invaluable to us. Going to meetings while I was pregnant made all the difference. (Call 880-LaLeche to find the moms' group nearest you.)

Sherri, mother of Emma, age 3½
New York

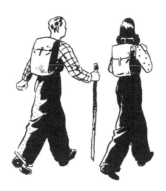

— Changing Relationships —

Sometimes the people you socialized with before having a baby now have little in common with you, or possibly they smoke or have other habits that you are not sure you want around your newborn. Don't burn bridges, but definitely build some new ones! Join a Moms club! It can especially help new moms. It's one of the best things I did for myself and my children!

Ann, mother of Billy, age 3, and Macy, age 1
Florida

Always be prepared for your youngest child to look like he/she has grown 6 inches since you gave birth to your newborn.

Misty, homemaker and mother of
Troy, age 9, Tiarra, age 7, Alexis, age 5, and Emily, age 3
Oklahoma

I know that the entire process of pregnancy, birth, and the first year will make you see your husband in a new light and fall in love with him in all different ways all over again, especially when he holds, kisses, and talks to your baby.

Lea, courtesy of The Center for Conscious Parenting, www.cfcp.info, mother of
two little gems ages 3 and 2½ months
Oregon

Like most women in American, I went through my teens and the first half of my twenties with a very poor body image. I swallowed society's messages hook, line, and sinker and was very focused on how my body looked rather than how it functioned. Therefore, I approached the whole concept of getting pregnant with a lot of doubt. I deeply desired to have a baby, but I didn't trust my body. I was afraid that I'd have fertility problems or miscarriages or horrible, painful labors. I expected that my body would let me down in this important area of life, just as I believed at the time that my body had let me down in other ways.

None of these fears came true. I had no problem getting pregnant twice in my twenties. My morning sickness was manageable, I didn't have a miscarriage, and I had no weird symptoms or complications during either pregnancy. I loved the feeling of being pregnant; of knowing that my body was doing something mysterious and wonderful; of feeling the baby move and get heavier and be my little companion day and night. After two full-term pregnancies, I gave birth to nine-pound babies with only one dose of Dermerol for pain each time. My body came through with flying colors in an area of functioning that was supremely important to me.

Breastfeeding worked like a charm also. My milk came in on schedule, my babies had no problem latching on; the milk just let down like it was supposed to, and it was incredibly affirming to watch my babies grow beautiful and strong, still nourished by my body.

Pregnancy, birth, and breastfeeding not only gave me two wonderful children, but gave me a different perspective on living inside a body that I had hated and resented for years. All of a sudden, I had a whole new way of looking at my belly and my breasts. "I may think this sticks out too much," I thought, "but inside that belly my body parts really know what to do. These breasts of mine have seemed too small all of my life, but they sure can produce a lot of milk!"

Becoming a mother created a turning point in my relationship with my body. While it didn't cure me of all my body image issues (at age 42, I still struggle in this area sometimes), motherhood helped me make friends with my body. Fertility, gestation, birth, and breastfeeding are functions that millions of years of evolution have designed our female bodies to accomplish. We women need to look at our bodies in the context of these functions and claim them as a tremendous source of strength and specialness in our lives.

Motherhood helps me fight society's messages that appearance is where it's at and feel grateful for all the things my body can DO and do well. If you open yourself emotionally to the mystery and joy of every step in the process, motherhood can do the same for you.

**Jocelyn Miller, Ph.D., child psychologist and mother of
Keaton, age 17, and Danneka, age 14
Wisconsin**

We live with mothers our whole lives. By the time we become young adults we think we know them. We feel certain that we know what makes them tick and that we have even figured out what makes them cry for seemingly no reason. Beyond that, we believe we know what they know, have been where they have been, and that we have seen all that they have seen.

When we become adults, we think that we have finally realized what it means to have a deep-seated, genuine appreciation and affection for our mothers, and we think that we are truly thankful for everything they have ever done for us. And then, we get pregnant.

For nine solid months complete strangers are hurling unsolicited advice at us about everything from hemorrhoids to breastfeeding. We listen intently as they describe in graphic detail the horrors of childbirth, infant shots, and baby bowel movements until one precious and glorious moment when our lives come full circle, and we stand firmly on the foundation that our very own mother passed down to us. It is only at that moment when we first become mothers ourselves, that we finally realize that the story began not with birth, but in the exact instant that our mother's womb was used to conceive of our very life. The realization that every breath and priceless memory we have is the culmination of her choices in life can be humbling and overwhelming.

When I became a mother myself I realized that this kind and gentle person who loved me so dearly and who knew everything about me had been a complete stranger for all these years; not because I did not bother to try and understand her, but because I couldn't understand her the way I do now that I am a mom, too. Pregnancy changes more than just your body: it changes your heart, your hope, and your future. Every relationship you have will be different after you have children.

Brandi, advertising and mother of Tyler, age 1
Georgia

As a mother of seven sons, I have learned to live by a simple credo…"Everyone gets what they need and SOME of what they want." That means if a child wants to go to the park but his little brother needs a nap, we stay home for the nap, and big brother can play in the backyard. If baby needs to nurse frequently and mother needs to sleep more, we find a way for both ends to be met. If parents sacrifice everything, they will burn out. If kids get everything, they will be self-centered. Everyone must learn to identify needs versus wants, and then the parents should teach the children to prioritize accordingly without complaining.

Grace, childbirth educator, doula, and mother of Logan, age 14, Jeremy, age 11, Ian, age 8, Sean, age 5, Quin, age 4, Duncan, age 4, and Samuel, age 1
Maryland

Get a babysitter very soon! You need to get out either alone, with your husband, or with a friend. And the earlier you begin with this, the easier the baby will adjust to other caregivers. Don't worry about the cost: a) you can't afford not to take care of yourself and your marriage (You were a woman, wife and friend before the baby came and you will be long after they leave.) and b) there are PLENTY of women, for instance, who would love to hold and cuddle a baby for a couple hours while you get a much-needed break...use them!

Courtesy of the moms of Blackberry Creek Community Church in Aurora, IL

Try to have a regular "date night' with your spouse: no kids and no kid talk allowed. Make it only the two of you. This will help refresh and reinvigorate new life into your relationship. I've also found that when I have time away from my kids, time to be a "grown-up," I am a better mother when I am with them.

Mindee, mother of Daniel, age 3, and Eitan, age 1
Missouri

Be prepared for constant adjustments that need to be made as new parents. Having a baby really creates a whole new reality, and it is not just about who does what and when. Be prepared to have to make time to talk, to check-in, to hand-off the baby, to absorb frustration according to the needs of your partner. Communication takes on a whole new importance. You must not underestimate how important it will be to talk and discuss feelings, schedules, fears, frustrations, joys, etc. In some ways you and your partner have never been more different. You will approach situations differently — one way is not necessarily the right way. It is common in our society for men to be critized for their parenting. Don't be arrogant just because you are the mom. Try to be unselfish in sharing your baby with your partner. (This is easier for some of us, harder for others.) Talk, talk, talk. You may exchange harsh words of frustration in the heat of the moment, but make sure to always come back and talk it out when you have some time. This is especially important advice for those folks who have been together for a long time. Your relationship is about to change: you can make it for the better.

The contributing moms of "The List," a growing list of
new mom tips passed from friend to friend
New Jersey, Maryland, and Delaware

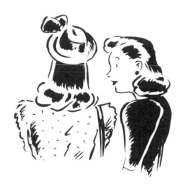

─Fighting Isolation─

Try to find a local support group for MOMS and children. It is a GREAT way to get to know other moms and to talk about all your motherhood struggles and achievements. Plus, it's a wonderful way for your children to make new friends and develop social skills. I am currently the president of such a club, and it has been so beneficial to both me and my two children.

Ramanda, stay-at-home mother of Wesson, age 4½, and Gracie, age 8 months
Arkansas

JOIN a group — any group — for yourself and for your child's socialization.

Tara, high school teacher and at-home-mother of Kiley, age 2
California

After Ethan was born, I nearly went into isolation mode. Luckily, my mom and sisters forced me out. This actually gave me more energy and kept me from feeling depressed. Don't over do it, of course, but go out grocery shopping, for coffee, etc. The more you go out, the better you'll feel!

Kristi, technical support and mother of Ethan, age 5 months
Washington

Talk to other mothers about what parenting is REALLY like. Discuss your fears and frustrations unabashedly. Don't sugarcoat life as a mama when speaking to other parents. Most importantly, find a community of honest, loving parents – seek their advice and share experiences. Be humble, acknowledge that no one will ever be a perfect parent, and have confidence in yourself and your parenting skills.

Kristina, registered nurse, LDPR, and mother of
Hannah, age 5, and Annabelle, age 1 month
Rhode Island

Nowadays few of us live near our mothers, aunts, sisters, cousins, and grandmothers. We need to create a network of women who will support us as mothers, women with whom we can be ourselves. Mothering is hard work, and we need to let off steam and share ideas with a safe group. My favorite support has always been La Leche League. Find your local group and see if you agree!

Stephanie, mother of Kate, age 8, and Ben, age 6
Maryland

Build a support network. Ask for help and allow yourself to be helped and contributed to. Recruit friends, family, neighbors, bosses, your work colleagues, and professionals to be available as needed. Maintain contact with your network and always have backup and emergency plans! Create harmony in your life — a mixture of work, family, and friends. Remember, there is no single formula for balance. How you combine your spouse, children, and career is a personal process.

Natalie Gahrmann, author of *Succeeding as a SuperBusy Parent*, life and parent
coach, and mother of two
New Jersey

Moms groups are a great way to get out of the house with your baby and meet the social needs of both you and your child. Hospital and park district groups, exercise classes, and baby music classes are just a few of the many places that may facilitate moms groups. Many groups offer educational speakers in the parent field, too. Some of your future friends-for-life will be met in these new places!

Courtesy of ParentPrep, parent educators
Illinois

Get connected! Whether pregnant or a new mom, finding other moms with whom you can connect is so important for your own sanity as a mom and for learning more about parenting from others. Especially for new moms, it's often hard to know what is "normal" or common with other children and how to handle issues, despite the wealth of parenting books out there. Find moms in your neighborhood or community who can share their knowledge, expertise, and resources. You will feel less isolated and learn some invaluable lessons!

Nancy, executive director of Holistic Moms Network and mother of Michael, age 3, and expecting in 2005
New Jersey

Be sure to get lots of support – people who believe you can be a great parent even when you have your doubts. YOU are the best parent for YOUR child. Find your way together.

Susan, Discovery Toys educational consultant and mother of Noah, age 5, and Isaac, age 1
Washington

Join an online community of moms. The MomExchange, www.momexchange.com, is the premier moms organization for mothers loving and raising newborn through teenage children. Our mission is to connect moms and give them opportunities to ask questions, build relationships, and get answers from other moms. The MomExchange is both an online and offline community of moms focused on connecting, collaborating, and educating moms just like you with information, resources, and discounts in an informative and fun way.

Gabrielle, media and marketing and mother of Jake, age 8, and Giavanna, age 6
California

Join a moms club. Visit www.momsclub.org.

Jessica, mother of Steven, age 6, Olivia, age 5, and George, age 2
New Jersey

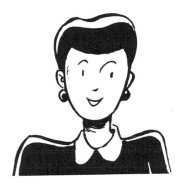

— Trusting Your Instincts —

You know your baby best! If you think something isn't right, and you have checked everything but sense your baby isn't being himself/herself – trust your instincts!

Dawn, mother of Elizabeth, age 9, Tabitha, age 8, William, age 5, and Abigail, age 1
Virginia

With any advice relating to raising your child, ask yourself, "Do I feel okay with this?" Whether it be regarding sleeping, feeding issues, daycare, discipline, etc. – if it doesn't feel right to you, listen to your instincts. You know your child better than anyone; and for every bit of advice, there is someone who will contradict that. Listen to the "words of wisdom," study the research, use what feels right for your family, and leave the rest.

Jacque, CLE and mother of Kyleigh, age 8, and Karissa, age 4½
California

Trust your instinct (I mean actively LISTEN; check in with it all day long!). It will tell you the right path to follow with each child.

Laura, mother of Brynn, age 14 months
Minnesota

There are so many opinions on parenting (professional and otherwise), but the best advice you can follow is your instinct. You know your child better than anyone else, so the best thing you can do for your child is what works best for the family.

Alisa, mother of Benjamin, age 5½, and Lucas, age 2½
Texas

The best advice I was given and proved invaluable to me was to trust my own feelings. If something just didn't seem right to me, I listened to my heart and was so much less stressed out.

Lynda, mother of Ernie, age 18 months
Florida

I think the only tip I want to share is trust yourself and your baby. It is so difficult to stay calm and trust ourselves in the middle of so much advice from so many different kinds of good people. When you add to it a difficult pregnancy, a high need baby, a sick baby, or sleepless nights, that is the perfect set up not to hear your heart and your baby. Nobody has a miracle recipe that works with everyone. You know best. Ask your heart, ask your baby, and you will get the answer you need.

Paloma, student midwife and doula and mother of
Yuri, age 6½, and Aysha, age 4½
Texas

Never forget that, by nature, mothers are overflowing with positive instincts that keep those beautiful babies and children of all ages safe. Always trust and read into your motherly instincts! My motherly instincts have, so far, prevented unnecessary medical procedures on my oldest son when he was three; saved the life of my middle son at birth; and allowed me to have the best and simply empowering natural water/homebirth with my youngest son.

Saraj, mother of Adam, age 11, Samantha, age 8, Breyley, age 5, and Anthony, age 3
Wisconsin

Trust your instincts – they are usually right.

Kara, mother of Kyle, age 11 months
New Jersey

Do what is best for you and your baby. I thought peer pressure was over, but I learned of a new kind called "parent peer pressure." Treasure every moment as you desire!

Amy Tardio, therapist, counselor, and mother of John, age 1
Illinois

Listen to your heart…you know what is best for your own child. Hold your baby and respond to your baby's cries.

Sherri, mother of Emma, age 3½
New York

No matter how many well-meaning people give you (solicited and unsolicited) advice on everything about raising your baby, trust your own instincts and know that YOU do know what is best for you, your baby, and your family.

Meg English, owner of Trimesters Boutique and mother of
Morgan, age 11, and Lawson, age 2
Pennsylvania

Advice on how to parent will come from everywhere. But the best place that perfect advice will come from is your intuition. Trust it, because it is never wrong.

Jessica, stay-at-home mother of Kenneth, age 2, and Nikara, age 8 months
Arizona

Don't read every article and book about baby stuff. Enjoy these first years and just go with your instinct. As a mother, your senses to your baby will be heightened and will tell you what NO book can.

Angela, homemaker and mother of Dylan, age 10, and Nicholas, age 1½
California

As a parent, follow your instincts! There are many "experts" out there. You and your child are unique. Do what you feel is best for your child, even if it goes against the norm. You are the expert. You are the momma!

Laura, mother of Nolan, age 14, and Neva, age 16 months
California

You will know instinctually how to take care of your child but will often second guess yourself because of poor advice from people who think they are helping you. Trust your intuition. It is your God given instinct to life. If you think the baby wants to be held, hold him/her. If you think the baby is hungry, nurse him/her. If you think that your baby is just over stimulated, you are probably right. Mothers truly know best.

Amanda, stay-at-home mother of Samantha Alexis, age 11 months
Ohio

Trust your instincts. If something doesn't seem right about your baby, do not be afraid to "bother" the doctor with it. My first child's doctor told me that motherly instinct is right more often than not. YOU are your baby's specialist, so to speak, the one who knows your baby the best.

Mara, La Leche League leader, counselor when employed, and stay-at-home mother of Gabrielle, age 4, and Alexander, age 1
Georgia

Always follow your intuition. Only you know your baby and his/her personality, needs, and wants. If you think something is wrong/right, it probably is. Nothing is stronger than your connection to your baby.

Cindy, mother of Caeley, age 6, and Cameron, age 4
California

It's important for moms to trust their instincts. Women receive so much advice when they are pregnant and even more once the baby is born. It's important for a family to do what they believe is best, even if it goes against advice they've been given. What works for one mom won't necessarily work for another. Women need to trust their maternal instinct.

Shelly, owner of www.munchkinmenus.com, and mother of Curtis, age 2½
Michigan

Follow your heart. If it feels right, it probably is.

Edit, veterinary technician and mother of Escher, age 3½ months
Ontario, Canada

Trust YOUR instincts. Most questions are "management," not "medical." Management questions elicit opinions from everyone (MD's, RN's, relatives, friends, etc.). Do what your baby and heart lead you to do. Remember, babies miss the womb. They need closeness and attention, not discipline.

Vicki Honer, Lamaze childbirth educator; international board certified lactation consultant, and mother of 3 adult daughters
Virginia

When there are behavioral problems — a child who is not sleeping well, screaming and crying all night — doctors or other well-meaning people have lots of advice, often saying that you should just let him/her cry it out or that the child is just trying to manipulate you. When they say there is nothing wrong with him/her, yet he/she is in obvious discomfort (i.e., stomach pain) and nothing seems to help, go with your gut and keep seeking additional opinions. It may be a food allergy or food sensitivity. Doctors are only now finding that there are food allergies that affect the intestinal tract but don't show up on normal skin tests, which was the case for my son. He has always had stomach problems (projectile spit ups as an infant; "sensitive gag" as a baby, toddler, and up to age 5; vomiting anywhere from daily to a couple of times a week; choking on his mucous during a tantrum, etc). There was something wrong, and I always knew it, but it took 6 years to finally confirm it. Thank goodness we live where we do, or we still wouldn't know. Children's Hospital of Philadelphia is one of only two hospitals in the country, that I know of, that do the Patch test that he had done, which is what confirmed the food allergies that affect his GI tract. So many parents just go with what the pediatricians or well-meaning family members are saying, and it takes so long to diagnose real problems. I've found out from other parents of food allergic kids that this is a common problem. If your instincts tell you there is a physical problem, they may be right.

Debbie, owner of www.coconutbeach.com, and mother of
CJ, age 6½, and Rachel, age 2
New Jersey

Many "experts" will give you all kinds of conflicting advice on parenting and how to raise your child. However, YOU are the only real expert on your child. Follow your own inner guidance on what is right for you, your child, and your family.

Marla, teacher and mother of Nikhil, age 6
Georgia

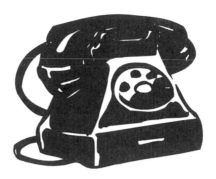

Advice

When people try to tell you that picking up a crying baby will spoil him/her, please don't listen. A crying baby needs to feel safe. Pick him/her up!

Karen, secretary and mother of Jeffrey, age 33, and Lori, age 30
Rhode Island

Absolutely everyone has an opinion about how you should handle sleep issues with your new baby. The danger to a new parent is that these tidbits of misguided advice (no matter how well-intentioned) can truly have a negative effect on our parenting skills and, by extension, our babies' development…if we are not aware of the facts. The more knowledge you have the less likely that other people will make you doubt your parenting decisions.

When you have your facts straight, and when you have a parenting plan, you will be able to respond with confidence to those who are well-meaning but offering contrary or incorrect advice. So, your first step is to get smart! Know what you are doing, and know why you are doing it. Read books and magazines, attend classes or support groups – it all helps.

Elizabeth Pantley, author of *The No-Cry Sleep Solution: Gentle Ways to Help Your Baby Sleep Through the Night* (Excerpted with permission by McGraw-Hill/Contemporary Publishing. www.pantley.com/elizabeth) and mother of Angela 17, Vanessa 15, David 14 and Coleton 5
Washington

You'll get advice from everyone under the sun, but do what works for you. Remembering the slogan "whatever works" has helped me justify letting my baby sleep with me, breastfeeding beyond a year, and other issues that everyone wants to give me advice about. Whatever works for you is what's best!

Wendy, stay-at-home mother of Tyler, age 8, and Alyssa, age 1
Colorado

As a parent and educator, I've observed the challenges that face new parents with every choice regarding their child's welfare. As parents soon discover, there are "experts" on every issue or concern. My tip: after you've reviewed all the evidence, remember to check with your heart and intuition. Choose. Now, be at peace with your choice. This is the only way to stay sane. There will be an equally important choice just ahead of you so there's no time to run yourself down with second guesses.

Jesse, childbirth educator, birth doula, and mother of Dashiell, age 1
Oregon

My tip for the first year is this: RELAX. It will only get easier! You may feel completely exhausted through lack of sleep and being on the go 24/7; you may feel that everyone else knows better and that you must be doing something wrong. Everyone else knows why your baby won't stop crying — he's hungry, tired, too hot, too cold, it's windy, etc., but it doesn't matter. I found that with Kara (my first) I must have been doing it wrong, because everyone else always had an answer. But once I learned to just nod and smile and let well meaning advice brush by me and do what I thought was right (which became easier with each one!), I felt more relaxed and happy; and it almost became humorous. Be calm, relax whenever you can, and take it all in stride. Ask for help when you need it. Listen to what others have to say and take it all in and decide what to keep, using your own wisdom, knowledge, and common sense. Who cares what your mother-in-law, mother, or the lady across the street thinks? Smile inside...you have a lovely baby; this stage won't last forever.

Nanette, teacher and mother of
Kara, age 9, Zoe, age 7, Jed, age 6, and Dom, age 2
London, United Kingdom

Read books and listen to advice, but in the end, remember YOU are the mother, so follow your instincts. And, of course, listen to advice with a smile – you might need that person as a babysitter later!

Cathy, mother of five, ages 10 to 2
Texas

If you are feeling low because other moms are telling you that you are not up to snuff in your parenting abilities, research some child rearing practices in other countries. You'll find that some entire cultures do it your way, and it will encourage you that your child will be okay just like the children in the culture that follows practices similar to your own.

Kristi, therapist and mother of Zoe, age 15 months
Texas

Remember that the so-called experts do not live in your house or know your child. Always do what YOU think is best for your child and family – not just what the "experts" advise you to do at each stage! Also, remember that there are lots and lots of books available to help parents in their child rearing endeavors. The problem is that YOUR child hasn't read them yet!

Claudia, educator and mother of Taylor, age 4, and stepmother of
Austin, age 14, Saige, age 11, and Rylan, age 8
Tennessee

Don't let other people's opinions affect you. When I told people I was planning on cloth diapering, I got a lot of flack. Same for extended breastfeeding. Do what you feel is best for your situation and for your baby. If you get caught up in other people's opinions, you'll lose your own sense of intuition.

Julie, purchasing manager, Chinaberry Inc., www.chinaberry.com,
and mother of two
California

Try to get all the information you can about nursing your baby early in your pregnancy, and never take nursing advice from someone who failed at it.

Heather, registered nurse
South Carolina

As a first time mother, I sought out and received a lot of advice about what to do during pregnancy and for the first year, how to do it, and what were the wrong (!) things to do. I began to get nervous with so much input, and I found myself second-guessing my choices at all turns. After awhile I learned to get off the internet, turn off the television, and close the books. I realized I instinctively already knew how to handle it all if I just listened, believed my inner voice, and followed the cues that my little one was telling me from the beginning. I have been complimented many times on how well adjusted my little girl is; and every time I am asked how I did it, I can only say "I played it by ear." Everybody is different, and every child is special and has his/her own needs. So really, my best advice is to stop listening to advice! Your body till tell you what it needs when you are pregnant, and your baby will make it clear what his/her needs are. Nature is wonderful that way. So trust in your intuition, be flexible, and don't kill yourself if everything is not going as planned. Trust me, it never will, but you will always be the best mother for your child.

Renee, Web designer and stay-at-home mother of Alexandria, age 2
California

Have people write their advice, tips, and tricks on recipe cards. You can store them in a recipe box and choose to use them or not, and no one's feelings will be hurt, You won't get overwhelmed, and what an amazing collection of wisdom at your fingertips!

Micheline, doula, childbirth educator, lactation consultant, day care provider,
and mother of 3
British Columbia, Canada

If you have had a baby, you know that everyone comes out of the woodwork to tell you what you have to do, what works best, and what worked for their sister's cousin's best friend's sister-in-law. The best advice is don't listen to everyone else's advice! Follow your heart and trust in yourself and your abilities. Once you can remove all the advice from everyone that is cluttering your head, you can feel your natural instincts take over. Know that you are a wonderful mother doing what is best for you and your children.

Laila, work-at-home business consultant and mother of
Maria, age 2, and Matthew, age 4 months
British Columbia, Canada

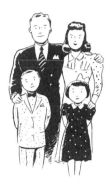

Parenting Styles

A mother's role is to teach her children right from wrong and to keep them from harm. A wise woman feels content because she has prepared her children to experience life on their own, and she knows that experience is the best teacher. A loving mother will always be available for her children with open arms to wipe away their tears when her children feel the stings of life.

Charlotte Du Brier, author of *How Not to be a Frazzled Bride* and mother of Marc David
Pennsylvania

Start as you intend to end. Don't teach your baby to go to sleep while bouncing in your arms if you're hoping he/she will learn to sleep by being still in the crib. In all aspects of motherhood, think about what you want your baby to learn and then start from there.

Lisa Druxman, CFM Chief Founding Mother Stroller Strides ™ and mother
California

Parenting trends come and go, but you'll never go wrong if you listen to your heart when parenting your child (even if your choice is not popular).

Melody, childbirth educator and mother of William, age 20 months
Virginia

Children always model their parents' behavior. It is what they see most. Therefore, being a calm and patient role model (though, not always easy!) will definitely help your children be calm and patient individuals.

**Denise, music teacher and mother of
Carina, age 7, Cecilia, age 5, and Isabella, age 1
California**

If I have learned anything, it is to be consistent. Decide what you want to accomplish in your child, then go about accomplishing it. Each day have your goal in the forefront of your mind – don't aimlessly raise your child. Start off right! Let your child know that you are predictable. Be consistent in scheduling your baby; discipline; playing together and independently; in your physical touch and affection to them and their daddy; and most of all in praying as a family and as an individual for your family. If you want your child to eat veggies, give him veggies *from the beginning*. If you want him to drink lots of water, give him water *from the beginning*. It is easy to do anything "right" *from the beginning*. Your young child only knows and experiences what you present him. It is difficult changing set habits or customs when he is older.

**Elisabeth K. Corcoran, author of
Calm in my Chaos: Encouragement for a Mom's Weary Soul (Kregel Publications,
www.kregel.com), and mother to Sarah, age 7½, and Jack, age 6
Illinois**

I keep getting asked by other parents, "What type of parenting style do you follow?" whenever they see my son and how happy he is. I answer back with "Instinctual; my heart. It didn't fail the human race thousands of years ago, and it won't fail me now." When parents ask what they should do, I also tell them to do what their heart tells them to do. If your baby cries out for you and your heart aches to pick him up, do it. It's that simple.

**Michele, SAHM, doula, lay midwife, childbirth educator,
and mother of Elijah Uriel, age 1
Oklahoma**

Don't sweat the small stuff. And remember…it's all just small stuff.

**Liz Wolk, RetroParents.com, and mother of Sam, age 10, and Eli, age 5
Washington**

Read Dr. Sears and read about attachment parenting! His child and parent centered wisdom is superb, and the attachment philosophy is a wonderful gift to baby and family.

Sherri, mother of Emma, age 3½
New York

The old adage "mothers know best" is probably the best advice that can be given to any new mother. For instance, it's true that breast is best but not to the detriment of mom's own health or sanity! When having a child for the first time, most mothers take anything they are told literally. Fashions have changed over the centuries. All children are different and will not need the same things.

Davina, housewife and mother of Felix, age 7, Cecily, age 5, and Jemima, age 2

Love, patience, consistency, and humor equal the making of wonderful parents and wonderful children.

Kathy, mother of Sophie, age 3
Nova Scotia, Canada

There are three things a parent/caregiver shouldn't mess (try to control, interfere) with: 1. Eating 2. Sleeping 3. Going potty. These are issues that can come back and resurface in many forms later in life.

Renee, store owner, La Leche League leader, and mother of
Ignacia, age 12, Ilexis, age 7, Ilia, age 6, Isaiah, age 2, and Isis, age 7 days
California

Take it as a compliment when people say that you are spoiling your child. Although spoiling really means "left alone to go bad," when used in context of a child, it means that the child knows 24/7 that he/she is loved.

Amanda, stay-at-home mother of Samantha Alexis, age 11 months
Ohio

Meeting your baby's nighttime needs is more practical, as well as more loving, than trying to persuade an infant about what he/she really needs.

Jo-Anne, mother of seven, stepmother of two,
and step-nanny of four living and two angels
Canada

My sister and her family were huge co-sleepers – everyone in one big bed. Even with 4- and 6-year-olds, they often sleep together. I thought "NO WAY!" until our son was born. Truthfully, we didn't co-sleep often, but there were many nights when he came to bed with us, or came back to bed after nursing, or slept the morning away with Daddy. What I realized is that there is no hard and true method. Don't discount a practice simply because it seems odd or unconventional at first glance. If it works for your family, it's a winner!

Melina, strategic workforce planning consultant and mother of Sebastian, age 2¾

All those times you said, "When I have a kid, I'll never…" or "My child will NEVER…" These, my friend, will come back to bite you right SMACK in the hiney! I promise!

Tina, bookkeeper and mother of
Fisher, age 5, Eli, age 2, and Sullivan, age 9 months
Texas

I never considered co-sleeping before our first child was born. I thought it was unsafe for the child, because I was raised by parents who thought that babies needed cribs from the first day they were home. I thought it was bound to lead to a 6-year-old sleeping with my husband and me and to the end of my relationship with my husband. I found out how wrong I was one night when we were both tired of getting up and lying down every hour or so when our newborn wanted to nurse more often than we ever anticipated. From that night on through the first few months of her life, it saved my husband and me a lot of trouble to have her in the bed with us so I could feed her when she woke during the night. It was less jarring to all of us. She didn't need to awake hungry and cry until one of us picked her up, and my husband and I didn't need to get out of bed. Everyone seemed to enjoy the closeness it brought, and when she began moving around more at night and seemed ready for her own bed, the transition was smooth. I look back now and laugh at all the comments we received from well-meaning people who thought that no good could come from letting our baby sleep with us. Now I cherish those memories of waking up next to her and being able to cuddle with her and my husband in the morning. Babies grow up way too quickly to worry about what other people think about you and your parenting those first few months. Enjoy the closeness and do whatever comes naturally!

Sarah , work-from-home tech writer and mother of
Juliana, age 15 months
Illinois

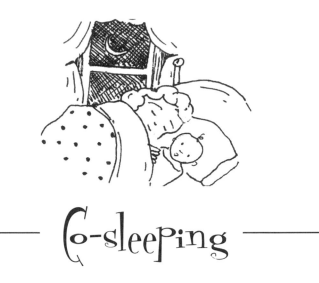

(o-sleeping

My husband and I decided that we wanted to share our bed with our daughter. (She was still in the orphanage at that time.) We understood fully that she did not get held as often as other children, and we wanted to instill a sense of security in her as well as catch her up for what she lost in her first year. She still needs us to fall asleep at 5 years old and then sleeps through most of the night alone. I have always loved sleeping next to her, and the best is taking a nap with her in the afternoon! We use her birthdays as milestones for the next stages in her developing her independence.

**Melissa, interfaith minister and mother of Annamika, age 5
Pennsylvania**

Try not to keep your baby in your bed at night past the age of 8 months. It is very difficult to rid baby of this habit if you continue to allow him/her to sleep with you. Just answer this question…"Do I want my child sleeping in my bed five years from now?" I bet the answer is "No!".

**Robyn, mother of Matthew, age 6, Devin, age 5, and Marissa, age 2
Pennsylvania**

Co-sleep and learn how to nurse lying down. It will save you hours of lost sleep and is a wonderful bonding experience, particularly if mom works.

**Claire, mother of Ellie, age 2
Arizona**

Don't be afraid to put baby in your bed! It's very safe as long as you haven't taken drugs, drank alcohol, smoked, are obese, or sleep on a waterbed. And it makes nighttime parenting SO much easier! Baby cries less since he's right next to Mama, and when he's hungry, you can sleep while he nurses! I can't imagine what it must be like for parents whose babies are in a separate room. They must be EXHAUSTED from getting up out of the bed so many times during the night! And take note — SIDS rates are actually much less among co-sleeping families. There's a reason that 90% of the world's population sleeps with their babies.

Sarah , stay-at-home mother of Adam, age 3, and Baby #2 due February 2005
Oklahoma

Something I wish I did from the beginning is co-sleeping. I did it one night when I was really tired and loved it. This helped me and my baby sleep better. I was able to meet her needs right away and better knew what she needed. She slept so well and woke up less. It was so easy to just nurse her right back to sleep, and most of the time I feel back to sleep with her. I loved waking up to her snuggled into me and happy! What a blessing to be able to tend to her so easily. Really, the thought of having a baby in another room altogether doesn't really make much sense. What a better way to know if your baby is okay: you just open your eyes for two seconds and peek at her sweet little face.

Lisa, stay-at-home mother of Abby, age 10 months
South Carolina

Co-sleep? Just do it! I was told so many times that I was creating such a bad habit by letting my daughter sleep with us, but it truly was the only way for any of us to get any sleep. Besides, even adults prefer to sleep next to the warm body of a person they love. Shouldn't a tiny, helpless baby, too?

Amanda, stay-at-home mother of Samantha Alexis, age 11 months
Ohio

Sleep whenever you can and, of course, prepare to sleep with your baby for as many years as it is mutually sane to do so. Have fun about when and where in your house you make love (other than your bed).

Meladee, courtesy of The Center for Conscious Parenting, www.cfcp.info, teacher
who is currently a very happy stay-at-home mother of
Colin, age 5½, and Rory, age 11 months
Oregon

By the time I had my third child I realized that the most exhausting part of mothering is not getting enough rest. The solution for me was to keep my baby right beside me in bed so that I didn't have to get up and down during those fussy periods in the night. Lack of sleep never became an issue, and it was so much better for all family members. It was a win-win situation.

Maureen
Vancouver, Canada

A new mom's biggest problem has to be getting enough sleep – an impossible task with a newborn in the house. Here is a big secret: co-sleeping will make your life so much easier! You simply roll over to nurse your baby when baby awakes. You don't even need to sit up to change a diaper. Then you can snuggle back to sleep much more easily than if you had to get up, make a bottle, retrieve baby from the crib, etc. Breastfeed and co-sleep and make your life so much easier! Moms and babies have done it for all of time. Simply make sure you take the safety precautions: the amount of space between wall/crib rail should be minimal, no soft bedding, minimal amount of blankets and pillows needed. Be safe and cautious and enjoy this wonderful time. My fondest memories are of my babies throwing their arms around my neck or shoulders in their sleep.

Kim, full-time mother of Tristen, age 3, and Josie, age 4 months
California

By the time my third child was born, I had it down. He slept with my husband and me, and I never did get that new mother fog! Every night I would put a changing cloth on top of the blankets on the bed. I had a friend make a wooden side rail so that our baby could not fall out. Just on the inside of that, I put a wipe warmer, diapers, tissues, "booger ball" – everything I might need during the night (also water on the night stand). When my baby awoke, I would nurse him, sit him up to burp, then sit up to change him – all I had to do was lay him down on the changing cloth in front of me on the bed. I used warm wipes for his comfort, tossed the soiled diaper in the basket right next to the bed, and laid down for another session of nursing. We both fell asleep, and I ended up getting much more sleep because I never got out of bed!

Amy, full-time mother of Abby, age 8, Nico, age 3, and Alex, age 1
Colorado

You should co-sleep with your baby. It makes nursing at night sooo much easier. It is easy to check on the baby, too: you just reach out your hand and touch him, feeling his breaths.

Sarah, civil engineer and mother of a little boy, age 2½
New York

Sleep with your baby! I've slept with all three of my kids, and I've never had the exhaustion that so many other mothers have, especially in those early weeks. And no, they don't stay in bed with you forever.

Amy, homemaker and mother of
Joshua, age 6, Jesse, age 4, Grace, age 2, and another on the way
South Carolina

I have found that sleeping with my babies helped them, in the long run, to sleep better at night. I slept with all of my children, and it is rare for us to have a sleepless night in this house. They all sleep in their own beds now. Sleeping with your children teaches them the security of knowing that you are there for them and that you will be there for them if they wake up and they are scared. In the long run they end up waking up less because they are comfortable knowing that you will be there when they wake up. Eventually we just moved them to their own beds with no transition problems.

Angela, stay-at-home mother of Brittany, age 11, Gabrielle, age 10,
Kassandra, age 7, Isabela, age 5, and Danijela 1
Virginia

Sleep with your baby! That makes nursing so much easier (just roll over and nurse!). Soon the baby becomes so efficient that baby will nurse and you won't even wake up! I was never tired when my son was a newborn because he slept with me!

Meena
Delaware

When you sleep with you baby, your sleeping rhythms sync up, so as your baby starts to wake, so do you. It is much easier on you than being jolted awake from a deep sleep. You are less tired, and you can respond to your baby before he/she pushes the "I'm hungry" panic button.

Edit, veterinary technician and mother of Escher, age 3½ months
Ontario, Canada

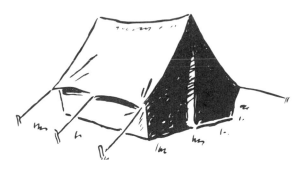

— Breastfeeding in Public —

Breastfeeding is such a wonderful experience for both mom and baby, but sometimes discretion is difficult. The second you covered my child's head with the blanket, he started grabbing at it or pulling off the breast. It's very difficult to feed a small tornado under a blanket. A trick from my mom: take the cover and fold it so it covers your bicep on the arm you are going to nurse the baby. Get baby in position and pull up your shirt, letting just a little more than the areola come out. When baby latches on, pull your T-shirt down over baby's cheek. Be sure when comfy to look up at someone or something – most people never even know I am feeding my child. If he pops off quickly, the T-shirt will fall down, and the blanket will cover the side view.

Mellissa, RN, and mother of Brennan, age 8 months.
South Carolina

Breastfeeding is economical, convenient, nutritional — very practical reasons for doing so. But I also found breastfeeding to be a very intimate action between me and my babies. Because of this treasured intimacy, I desired a certain amount of privacy and was selective when it came to nursing in public. Today's moms are much more mobile than I was as a nursing mom, and this mobility necessitates nursing in public. Finding a private area in a public venue may take some planning and/or creativity. Pick a spot where you will be comfortable both physically and mentally and baby will not be too distracted.

Joanne, editor and mother of four and grandmother of four
New Jersey

I know that sometimes nursing in public can be quite a hassle! I always bring a receiving blanket to cover myself while nursing. My blanket would always slip, and I found myself constantly readjusting. So I purchased a cute clothespin and pinned the blanket to my shirt. This helped make nursing much easier because I wasn't constantly putting the blanket back up.

Nicole, mother of Emma, age 2, and Ellie, age 2 months
California

Wear your baby, get out, and experience the world! A baby sling or front carrier is a great way to keep you and your baby happy. Your baby gets to be close and cuddly, and research supports that babies who are worn cry less and breastfeed more. What a great way to ensure that baby gets to nurse at least every two hours, while you get to see the world. It's easy to nurse in a sling, and many moms find they get so good at sling nursing, others can't even tell that your little one is having a snack as you sit at your favorite coffee shop or walk around the neighborhood. Slings are inexpensive and much easier to carry your baby in than most strollers. Just toss the sling on and go!

Beth, birth educator, doula, La Leche League leader, and mother of
Isaiah, age 4, and Noah, age 1½
Pennsylvania

Nurse your baby in public. It's so good to have other moms who may be considering breastfeeding to see another woman doing it in public. Know if there are laws in your state protecting breastfeeding and share them with anyone who questions you. As long as it's okay for babies to drink out of bottles in public, it should be all right for babies to breastfeed in public!

Emily
Oregon

Get a comfortable baby sling and have a friend who has experience in slinging a baby show you how to do it. Carrying a baby in a sling is so convenient. You can breastfeed ever so discreetly, do chores around the house, go shopping, and even care for older siblings…all with happy baby next to you!

Sandy, physical therapist and mother of Marika, age 4, and Haley, age 1
California

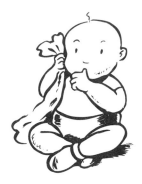

Enjoying the Moments

Hug them, love them, and enjoy them… they grow up so quickly!

The moms at Babygrams, Inc., www.babygrams.com

Try to let go of the little things and focus on growing a happy, healthy baby. Laundry and cleaning need to be done, but the baby is more important. They grow so fast – you won't want to miss a minute of it!

Mia, Web site owner/editor www.mainstreetmom.com, and mother of five, ages 9, 7, 5, 2, and "due November 2004"
Ohio

Relax. Everything passes – what seems like a huge emergency becomes an anecdote to be shared. The plus to having babies is that you and your baby will grow up together. Babies don't come with instruction booklets, and nature has figured out that their needs are small when babies are small and grow too as the babies grow up. This means you have the time to get acclimated. Above all, enjoy each phase – children are miraculous and each one has the right mom, just as each mom has the right child.

Karina, teacher and mother of Ben, age 18, and Ilana, age 16
Maryland

Whenever Megan needed "extra parenting" at night (translation: wanted me to lay next to her while she fell asleep), the following words repeated over and over again always helped me keep things in perspective, and even made her demanding request more of a joy than a resentment. "They are only little for such a short amount of time. Enjoy it ALL. It goes by so quickly."

Sheila, mother of Megan, age 29 months
Texas

Enjoy your baby. Count every freckle, memorize all of his facial expressions, kiss his little toes, listen to every coo and gurgle...in a few VERY short years, those melodic coos will transform into shrieks of "Mom! Stop staring at me!"

Deborah Shelton, author of
The Five Minute Parent: Fun & Fast Activities for You and Your Little Ones
and mother of Kizer, age 6

For me, one of the most surprising aspects of having a baby is how incredibly fast time goes. People will tell you how babies grow so fast and how the first year just flies by. But you can't really fathom what that means until you actually go through it. If I could repeat my baby's first year, I would relax more and enjoy each stage, even the difficult ones. I remember the first few months of nursing. Laura wanted to be at my breast every 20 minutes or more, and she would hang on for hours it seemed. The only time she ever nursed every three hours was at night. I hadn't expected this and was rather overwhelmed. I remember feeling very anxious because I had the idea that it would be like this forever. Then within a few months, Laura got more interested in the world around her and wouldn't nurse every time I offered her my breast. Gone were those wonderfully lazy days of lying in bed all day reading books and magazines or e-mailing all of my friends long letters while nursing my baby. I had actually begun to enjoy those hours of continuous nursing, and then just like that it was over, whether I was ready or not. So, whatever stage your baby is at, whatever it is you two are going through together, relax and go with it. Believe that it will end sooner than you think and you'll miss it. Laura is now one-year-old and starting to walk. She has this absolutely tender, sweet way of calling me "Mama" repeatedly, especially when she wants to nurse or just be with me. Ever time I hear her say "Mama," I want to burn it into my heart and remember it forever.

Fernanda, mother of Laura, age 1
Colorado

Risking sounding like a cliché, this time will not last forever. Begin training your mind and heart to freeze these special moments so you can bring them back to your memory when this baby gets bigger. When the words "Nothing can prepare you for a parenthood" finally make sense, ride this wave with gracefulness — it requires a lot of gratefulness. Sit back and enjoy the ride…it's a lot shorter than you think! Time flies when you're in love. Trust me.

Courtesy of the moms of Blackberry Creek Community Church in Aurora, IL

Be flexible and ready for anything. One day my two-year-old son was climbing on top of the kitchen table; I turned around, and he became 16 and is now driving a car.

Milynda, social worker and mother of Leif, age 16, and Mackinley, age 13
Michigan

When I find myself being overwhelmed by the fact that I would be responsible for my baby for the next 18+ years, I tell myself to take it day by day and to enjoy each precious moment because it flies!

Tracey, commercial real estate agent and mother of Brandon, age 10 months
California

First words are to have a sense of humor. The time as a new mom goes by so fast that although it seems like it will never end, it will be over before you know it. When it seems chaotic, just know you will survive and absorb this moment for what it is.

Lisa Druxman, CFM Chief Founding Mother of Stroller Strides™ and mother
California

Look for positives — there are so many! Enjoy every moment because the first year will fly by, even though you may not feel that way at the start! You'll look back at that first year with fond memories and wonder where it went. And that first smile, first roll, first crawl, first laugh, first word, first step…each will soon become harder and harder to remember! So relax, be confident, don't worry about anyone else's opinions, and enjoy your time with your baby!

Nanette, teacher and mother of
Kara, age 9, Zoe, age 7, Jed, age 6, and Dom, age 2
London, United Kingdom

They're growing up so quickly. Simply love them, love them, love them.

Lisa Mullane Viggiano, singer/songwriter and mother of David, age 2½
New Jersey

Smiles, cries, coos, boo-boos, hugs, kisses, no's, tiny toes…these are the best moments of the first year. Never forget it…this is the quickest passing year of your lives.

Tara, business manager and mother to Dylan, age 3, and Tyler, age 1
California

The first year does go as fast as everyone says, so do not sweat the small stuff — sleeping, how little baby eats, how quickly baby is developing compared to peers. Rather, spend that time and energy hugging, holding, and loving your child!

Alexandra, mother of Chloe, age 2 and expecting baby #2 in January
Pennsylvania

Hold your baby as much as you want to, for soon he/she will be leaping out of your arms.

Laura , mother of Brynn, age 14 months
Minnesota

Tired of all the crying, diaper changes, spit ups, and all the other unpleasantries of having a baby around? Just remember that it is for such a short time, really, as babies grow up so fast. Enjoy your baby as much as possible before the moment passes you by.

Kathy, mother of Sophie, age 3
Nova Scotia, Canada

Live in the moment. Look at your children today and enjoy who they are now. So often we are focused on lamenting about the past or planning for the future, forgetting that it's all about enjoying the right now.

Renee, store owner, La Leche League leader, and mother of
Ignacia, age 12, Ilexis, age 7, Ilia, age 6, Isaiah, age 2, and Isis, age 7 days
California

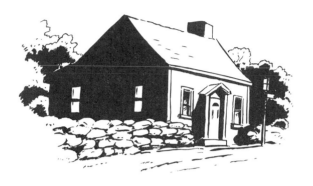

$\int$taying $\bigsqcup$ome

If you want to stay home and it looks like you can almost afford it, go for it. There are hidden costs associated with working, like transportation, clothing, and lunches, which add up. When I'm not working, I save money in lots of little ways. I plan meals and shop for groceries more carefully and eat leftovers for lunch. I also have time to find inexpensive or free entertainment. My big girl helps me wash the car so we can skip the car wash. I go over bills and have time to deal with them when I'm overcharged for something. Even if you save money in just a few ways that work for you, when you put all that together with the money you're not spending to work, it adds up to a significant amount.

**Kelly, psychotherapist and mother of Isabella and Wyatt
California**

If you choose to stay at home with your child, find a good support system of other like-minded people. I stayed at home with all four of my babies, and the most important thing was having a group of women around me who understood completely the innate desire to be with one's child during the early years. The bonding process between mother and child is intensified when they are together 24 hours a day. However, they do eventually pull away, but only when they are ready for it, and then they do so with such confidence.

**Maureen
Vancouver, Canada**

I highly recommend joining a moms group, especially if you choose to stay at home. For the first nine months of my daughter's life, I was isolated and lonely because I had quit my job, had no friends home during the day, and no stay-at-home moms in my neighborhood. I looked online and found a national mothers group called Mothers and More with a local chapter. I've been an active member for two years and have formed friendships with dozens of women with young children. I get out several times a week and credit this group with helping me postpartum with baby number two. I have not felt lonely or isolated; and when I feel blue or have a bad day, I have friends to cheer me up. I also recommend looking for stay-at-home moms at your church or place of worship. I have joined two other mothers groups, one at my local church. We have one playgroup each week, and the other meets bi-monthly for prayer and fellowship. My children are welcome at all of these activities and have also made many friends. Whether it be MOPS, Moms Club, the local library, YMCA, or some other group, I think that forming friendships with other mothers is invaluable.

Liza, stay-at-home mother of Anna Lucy, age 2, and Francis, age 8 weeks
Colorado

For me, there was no other option than to stay home with my son. Nothing else felt right. I was also very fortunate to have gotten laid off from my job, and the unemployment checks surely did help wean us off of my salary. However, staying home is not for everyone, and I think that it's really important that the decision be made without guilt. If you are used to living off of two salaries, it can be incredibly hard to adjust to just one. Start early. I have seen recommendations to bank one salary while living off the other. We just started to cut out whatever we could, knowing that my husband's salary was not enough to make me a kept woman. We stopped paying full price for everything, started buying and selling on eBay and other second-hand resources, and I took up some freelance work. It also helped to know that this situation was not forever; certainly, after a few formative years at home with the babies, we would not be opposed to having others care for them. For so many, returning to work is not a choice. But for those who do have the choice and make the choice, times may be a little tough, but there is no greater reward than days filled with baby smiles.

Kathleen , mother of Alejandro, age almost 3,
and twins Nieves and Paloma, age 9 months
New Jersey

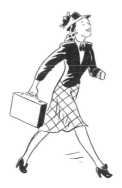

— Going Back to Work —

Instead of returning back to work on a Monday, ease back in by making Thursday or even Friday your first day back. It may feel less overwhelming for you to adjust to your new, busier morning routine for just a few days rather than an entire week.

Debbie, licensed clinical psychologist, founder of www.newsforparents.org, and mother of Emily, age 12, Ben, age 8, and Sam, age 2
Florida

Regardless of when you choose to return to work, it is often a difficult decision and one that requires some mental and emotional adjustments. Begin by assessing what you really want to do in your work life: What skills, talents, opportunities, and resources are available to you? What do you value? What do you need? Why do you want to work? What motivates and energizes you at work? You may decide to change careers or may have limited opportunities to pickup where you left off. You can pursue work in the same field, work related to a hobby, something totally different that you've always dreamed of doing. Using a gradual approach to prepare yourself emotionally, physically, and mentally will help smooth the transition.

Natalie Gahrmann, author of *Succeeding as a SuperBusy Parent*,
life and parent coach, and mother of two
New Jersey

Don't let family members, friends, or stay-at-home moms beat you up about going back to work. Not all of us get a choice. Cherish the time you do have; shut off the television. Don't get caught up in the righteousness that some stay-at-home moms have, and don't feel guilty if sometimes you enjoy going to work. Kids can sense love and happiness and will grow to understand the needs of a family.

**Katy, nurse and mother of Sean, age 18 months,
and expecting Baby #2 in March 2005
New Jersey**

Breastfeeding made easy for full-time career moms: When I had my son Logan, six years ago, my decision to breastfeed was easy to make. All the baby books, the free "advice" from experienced moms, the information in Lamaze classes – everything pointed to the clear advantages of breastfed babies over those only bottle-fed. The benefits were many: the baby would have a higher IQ, the mother would lose her pregnancy weight faster, the baby's dad would get a big fat pay raise to afford all of those diapers! (Okay, last one isn't actually documented but wouldn't that have been great?) The decision to breastfeed or not was the easiest of many things to come. Veteran moms did me right when they recommended the Medela double-breasted breast pump. It's pricey but well worth the investment. (After all, it is about to become your new best friend!) Purchase your breast pump early in your pregnancy and get to know how the system works. It is certainly not the time to be reading the instruction manual for the first time when your milk and baby arrive! Beside the pump itself, any mother returning to a full-time career should also buy a car adaptor that plugs into your cigarette lighter or auxiliary plug. Unless where you work happens to have a "Breastfeeding Lounge Area," (if so, I want to know where you work!), you'll be faced with locating a place to do your pumping while at work. Not an easy task! For me, the 5 x 5-inch, one stall women's bathroom at my office was not an option. What if I was all "hooked up" and some other woman suddenly came in to use the restroom? Fortunately, the car adaptor solved everything.

Each lunch hour, I would head for the parking garage located adjacent to our office building, plug the pump in, throw a blanket/afghan over myself, turn on the radio for some music, and read office mail/e-mail I never had time to read! As I headed out of the office each day, my boss (who was an older man with a sense of humor) called these time my "sabbaticals!" Other co-workers who weren't in on the "pumping process" must have thought that I had quite the "research" project going on out in the parking garage!

**Stacy, public relations and development coordinator of Eagle Village and mother of
Cassie, age 10½, and Logan, age 6
Michigan**

Don't let going back to work stop you from sharing the loving moments of breastfeeding for at least a year. At about 6 to 9 months, many children become more mobile and distracted when breastfeeding. Many mothers interpret that to mean their child is ready to wean. Quite to the contrary. Once they settle into their newfound activity level, they come back to the breast with vigor. Because breast milk is a natural anesthetic, you can help your child through shots, painful teething episodes, and bumps and bruises. Even more importantly, you can share warm personal moments that you will cherish for the rest of your life. There is nothing like a child snuggling next to you and looking up at you lovingly while receiving loving nourishment from "momma." All of this, plus reduced risk for breast cancer, ovarian cancer, lymphoma for you, and reduced risk of diabetes, obesity, and ear infections for your baby. No wonder breast milk is called the "perfect food"!

Marilyn, mother of Alexandra Nicole, age 19 months
(and still breastfeeding!)
California

Try to keep your options open if at all possible. Do you want to work part-time? Work at home? Be a stay-at-home mom? Until you actually have the baby, you don't know who your baby will be. Some babies easily fall into a schedule (or so I'm told), but some never do. Some are content and quiet for long periods, and others are "high need" and require constant attention. Your plans may clash with your baby's personality. Also, if you're a first-time mother, you don't know how you will feel about returning to work. You don't want to end up feeling trapped by an iron-clad commitment you made before the baby was born.

Beverly, editor and mother of Julia, age 24, and Eric, age 18
New Jersey

Just because you go back to work doesn't mean you have to stop breastfeeding. I pumped three times a day for 11 months before quitting my job to stay home. I am so thankful I stuck with it, even though I gave up my few minutes of free time at work. Now that it's all over, I feel so satisfied that my baby has been nourished by nothing artificial, and our breastfeeding relationship is still in tact. It was always a comfort to come home and reconnect with my baby as we rocked and nursed at night.

Amanda, stay-at-home mother of Samantha Alexis, age 11 months
Ohio

As a working mom, I thought the hassle of pumping and nursing would be more than I could handle. But I found that those times when I had to stop during the day and look at a picture of my little guy and think about him, combined with the utter bliss I felt when he was latched on at night or in the morning, were the best moments. I never was one to be a stay-at-home parent; it's just not in me. But to be able to share that bond with my child was worth every bit. He nursed until almost 12 months, and I wish it had been longer. I believe it – breast is best!

Melina, strategic workforce planning consultant and mother of Sebastian, age 2¾

If you've been breastfeeding your baby, it is well worth the efforts to continue after you return to work even though you'll be faced with many challenges. It will require commitment and work if you are determined to continue to breastfeed. If you want to continue breastfeeding after you return to work, you'll need to: choose a child care provider who supports your commitment to breastfeeding; establish a good milk supply so that you can more easily maintain it; select an appropriate breast pump; arrange breaks at regular intervals during the day in order to have time to pump (or feed your baby); arrange a comfortable private place to pump (preferably with an electric outlet); make use of lactation support services through your hospital or workplace; have a place to wash your breast pump after using it; arrange a suitable place to store your milk.

Natalie Gahrmann, author of *Succeeding as a SuperBusy Parent*,
life and parent coach, and mother of two
New Jersey

After a three month leave, it was very difficult to go back to a job that required quite a bit of travel. I continued to breastfeed via pumping (which I did in the airport bathroom, rental car, and many different office buildings!) which helped me feel like I was still providing for my baby when I was away. I also made sure I went to bed early when on the road and rested as much as possible when traveling to recoup from lost sleep from a no-sleeping baby when I was home! This saved my sanity and health.

Rebecca, insurance trainer and mother of Allye, age 13, and Addie, age 2
Texas

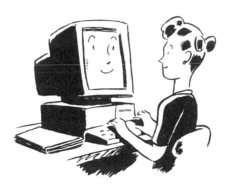

— Working from Home —

Know what you want from your home life and business life. Decide what is truly important to you and work towards that goal. If your priorities are in line, setting and achieving your goals is much easier because you are more focused on what is important.

Lesley Spencer, founder and director of HBWM.com, Inc - HomeBasedWorkingMoms.com Network
Texas

You can stay home with your kids and still earn money. Don't let someone else raise your kids. Be home with them everyday.

Shannon
North Carolina

Develop a schedule that allows you focused work time. Hire someone to come in during the week if you have children at home full time or consider part-time pre-school. Do not allow work to interfere with your children's needs. Strive for balance and remind yourself often what you want in life. If it's more time with your family, don't let your ambition interfere with your family's needs and time together

Lesley Spencer, founder and director of HBWM.com, Inc - HomeBasedWorkingMoms.com Network
Texas

Be aware of time-stealers. Ask yourself if this project, client, or task is beneficial for you, your business, and your family. If not, take steps to move away from it.

**Lesley Spencer, founder and director of HBWM.com, Inc -
HomeBasedWorkingMoms.com Network
Texas**

If you are planning on working at home without child care, think again and plan for help. I've worked at home for about 10 years so I thought working at home with a baby would be easy. And it was…for about 4 months…until my son's demands increased. I felt guilty for not spending enough time working and even worse about not spending enough time with him. At that point I realized I was being unrealistic, thinking that I could be a full-time mom and full-time business owner. My husband and I talked about it, and we made changes that made us both happy and, more importantly, made sure Holden was always getting the attention he needed. My husband always wanted to be an actor and had worked jobs that allowed him the freedom to go on frequent auditions. We decided that he would become a stay-at-home dad but would pursue acting opportunities as they arose. My mother-in-law agreed to baby-sit two days a week and to cover for my husband if an unexpected acting job came along. When Holden was about one year old, my father retired and started taking Holden on adventures one day a week. My mother works with me in the office and baby-sits on many weekends.

I think the results were well worth all the juggling. My husband has an incredible, hands-on relationship with our son (and his acting career is going great!). I spend everyday with my son and nursed him until he was one, built my business, and feel like I make an important contribution to our family. Holden's grandparents are an important and daily part of his life, and they really got to see him grow and thrive. We are all grateful for the opportunities we've had. It took some creative thinking and compromise and is an ever-changing process.

**Connie, publisher and mother of Holden, age 3
New Jersey**

Ask your spouse and older children to help out with the household chores and simple business tasks. Double your recipes and freeze meals for later use. Plan all of your errands for one day of the week.

**Lesley Spencer, founder and director of HBWM.com, Inc -
HomeBasedWorkingMoms.com Network
Texas**

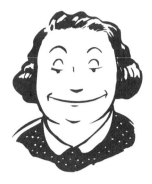

Finding Child Care

What to look for when hiring a NANNY.

1. Experience: Examine and explore work history (including child care), life experiences, and education.

2. Compatibility: Do you concur on child rearing and discipline philosophies and approaches? Are your habits similar? (i.e., neatness, organization, timeliness, flexibility vs. rigidity, food choices, priorities)

3. Qualities: Does the applicant have a natural inclination to connect to and understand the needs of children at each stage of development?

4. Common sense and patience: A nanny needs an extraordinary amount of both.

Wendy Sachs, president of The Philadelphia Nanny Network, Inc., and mother of Ross, age 14, and Bess, age 11

What to look for in an AGENCY.

1. Screening and background checking methods: Know specifically the depth of child care reference checks and applicant interviews.

2. Availability of agency personnel: Do you get an answering machine when you call or is there someone in the office during business hours?

3. Breadth of experience and reputation: If the agency has been in business a short time, expect them to be short on experience in

screening applicants and counseling on hiring a nanny. If the agency has been in business a long time, expect more experience in the ability to detect the more subtle red flags that only experience can define. Word of mouth reputation is important. Agency fee should reflect agency's expertise.

Wendy Sachs, president of The Philadelphia Nanny Network, Inc., and mother of Ross, age 14, and Bess, age 11

If hiring a NANNY on your own:

1. Ask DETAILS about background and work history since high school graduation.

2. Check ALL child care jobs and verify ALL employment.

3. Contract to do a state criminal check, DMV check, and social security number verification.

Wendy Sachs, president of The Philadelphia Nanny Network, Inc., and mother of Ross, age 14, and Bess, age 11

When choosing a day care, here are some things to look for that the books don't tell you: Are the caregivers on the floor with the children? (If they are, it means close interaction is going on.) Are there toys all over the place? (This tells you that a lot of fun is happening here.) And when touring the school with the director, do a lot of the kids come running up to him/her? (This tells you whether he/she is involved daily with the kids or locked up in the office.) Go with your gut feelings. Look beyond the building and the classroom. Who you are hiring are the people to love and care for your child. Trust your instinct about the environment!

**Harriet, retirement consultant and mother of
Garrett, age 3, and Isabella, age 16 months
California**

Go with your gut instinct...do the concrete, check references, driving record, work eligibility, do trial days. Even if that all seems positive and you do not have a good gut instinct, it is not the right fit. You will know when you have the right person. It is a different arena entirely, but I always tell my clients you will know it like your wedding dress...you just know.

**Robin LeGrand, A Nanny Corporation, Inc., and mother of Lake, age 10 months
California**

Nothing is more anxiety producing for a parent than hiring a stranger to care for your children. The anxiety level is understandably raised a notch when parents consider care by a nanny. It appears to be a greater "leap"…someone in your home, unsupervised, caring for your children.

So, how does a parent reduce the stress of hiring a nanny and feeling comfortable with the choice you make? The process of searching, interviewing, and hiring a caregiver should be the same as the process you would use to hire any employee. That is more easily said then done. A parent does not have the resources of a corporate HR department to make sure that all the "i's" are dotted and the "t's" are crossed. But if a parent takes the time and makes the effort, it can be done individually or, if not, in partnership with a professional nanny agency.

It is important to understand that you are searching for someone who will be a caregiver for your children, not someone who necessarily shares your interests. In addition to experience, location, age experience, requirements, hours, salary, and benefits, it is critical to evaluate and discuss the personality, lifestyle, childrearing philosophy, and "neatness quotient" of the caregiver. Develop a list of questions to ask EACH potential applicant…if you don't, they will all seem the same, or you might gravitate to someone because of her mannerisms versus her capabilities. Just because an applicant was referred by a coworker's sister versus responding to an ad in the newspaper does not mean the caregiver should receive less scrutiny. This is a mistake that many parents make. Characteristics such as strengths, weaknesses, future goals, hobbies, and interests are all very important. Require all applicants to bring a resume or timeline of employment (which includes dates, supervisors' names, and phone numbers) for the last 5 to 15 years (depending on their age).

The interview process should consist of at least two (preferably three) interviews. The first interview should not include the children. You are trying to decide if you even want to introduce this person to your children. The second interview is always at home and should be about two hours with all family members present. If you are still interested in pursuing the applicant, confirm phone numbers of references and tell the applicant you would require her to provide information necessary for you to do a criminal background check and Department of Motor Vehicles check (if she will drive your children). The applicant's name, address, date of birth, social security number, driving license number and state, and her signature (in some states) are required. If she hesitates or says no, you should rule her out as a potential candidate.

In addition, you should provide the applicant with the draft job description you completed and have a preliminary discussion about compensation expectations. Confirm that you will be checking the applicant's references. Encourage the applicant to call you if she has any questions and request that she call you before she accepts any other opportunities. Call her references and tell them that your discussion is confidential to encourage them to be completely honest in their comments. At a minimum ask about the applicant's creativity, dependability, strengths, weaknesses, self-esteem, why she left, would they rehire her, and her ability to communicate.

If your reference checks are successful, contact a private security company or nanny agency that provides nanny screening to perform the checks mentioned. If results are favorable, call the applicant to schedule a time to meet and make an employment offer and to review the job description. It is always best to give the applicant a day or two to review the job description and accept or negotiate the offer. If accepted, both you and your caregiver should sign the written job description as well as a summary of the financial terms of your offer. It is especially helpful to also include House Rules related to the job regarding petty cash, phone rules, where she can go (and not go), and what she can do with the children without asking for prior approval.

**Betty Davis, president and founder of In Search of Nanny, Inc.,
and mother of Allison, age 20, and Stephanie, age 17
Massachusetts**

Children are not born with a "How-To" manual, and nannies are not mindreaders. If the caregiver knows what you want BEFORE she begins work, you will have a much better chance of hiring a caregiver that will meet your expectations and provide the best care for your children. To start your process, you should:

· Define the characteristics, personality, education, and experience of potential caregivers you would consider.

· Describe your family and the interaction the caregiver will have with all family members.

· Describe your children's personalities, schedules, any special needs/medications and the priorities for each individual child for the next 6 to 12 months.

· Define the job, including what hours and flexibility you need and specific responsibilities.

· Describe the compensation you can offer and what benefits you might negotiate.

Once you complete the above, you are now ready for the next step. You have described your children and your expectations, your family, and the specific job requirements, and you know what you can afford to offer a caregiver.

**Betty Davis, president and founder of In Search of Nanny, Inc.,
and mother of Allison, age 20, and Stephanie, age 17
Massachusetts**

Put up a notice at a local seminary if available to find a local seminarian's wife to baby-sit. The wives are often times in their early twenties, have a college degree, and are living in a strange area while the husbands attend seminary. Their schedules are often more flexible (daytime and evening), and they are more responsible than most teenagers, which was the key with my twin babies.

Tara, mother of twins Caroline and Ryan, age 2½
Washington

Need some time off? Arrange alternating play dates with a friend. She'll take your kids, say, the first and third Monday afternoons of the month, and you'll watch hers on the second and fourth Mondays. Tip: Try not to giggle incessantly when you drop your kids off.

Jen Singer, author of *14 Hours 'Til Bedtime* and mother of
Nicholas, age 7, and Christopher, age 6
New Jersey

There are many benefits to using in-home child care. You don't have to get your children ready to go out every day or take them out in bad weather. You save time by eliminating drop offs and pick ups. Your children receive more personal attention than in a center with several others. Your children have the stability of remaining in the familiar environment of their own home. Your children's illnesses will not prevent them from attending day care so you take fewer days off work. Your child is exposed to much fewer viruses and is less likely to get sick as often as children in a day care setting. Your family gets the opportunity to form a lasting relationship with a caring person on whom you can depend. The family's schedule is more flexible since the nanny can drive them to their various activities. It is easier to monitor the care of you children in your own home. A nanny might be available beyond the typical hours of a center. A nanny might accompany the family and assist during travel or even spend overnights with the children while you are away. Parents who work from home can remain connected with their children easily without the risk of distraction from their job.

Amy Brixey, owner of The Nanny Option and mother of Kellen, age 16 months
Missour

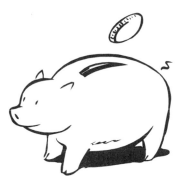

Money Matters

Begin a savings account for your baby immediately. When your friends and grandparents remember birthdays with gifts of money, add it to your regular contributions. You will be surprised how those little amounts can grow, too. What a pleasant surprise when it's time for college tuition.

Joanne Seymour, entrepreneur and author and mother of Dan, Mary, and Emily
Iowa

As a mom of four, I have always searched for ways to save money, especially when our children were very young. Using cloth diapers and making homemade diaper wipes saved us a bundle, as did shopping at garage sales in our local area as often as possible. It takes a little extra time to save money, but I promise you your efforts will be well rewarded. Enjoy this time with your baby; it's a blessing straight from heaven!

Michelle Jones, editor of BetterBudgeting.com, and GrocerySavingTips.com, and mother of Christine, age 14, Joshua, age 11, David, age 9, and Rachel, age 5
North Carolina

Consider forming or joining a baby-sitting cooperative to give yourself extra free time, spend time with other parents, save money on baby-sitting, and have your children enjoy time with friends.

Annmarie, attorney and mother of Eve, age 3, and Nathaniel, age 4 months
New Jersey

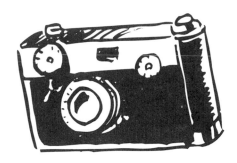

— Preserving Memories —

To help keep the many pictures of baby organized, buy a photo album for each year. On the inside cover write child's name, age, and the year. For example:

"John, 1-2 years old
March 1999-March 2000"

Then, as you get your pictures developed, just put them in order in the album. Be sure to write any pertinent information on the backs of the pictures!

Tanya, stay-at-home mother of Dennis, age 5, and Joseph, age 1
Florida

One of my biggest tips is that you can never have enough pictures... keep even those that don't come out well or you end up with copies of. Once that infant becomes a two/three-year-old, he/she will love having his/her very own copies of his/her pictures.

Abby, mother of Joey, age 7, Alyssa, age 5, Nicholas, age 3,
and Seth, age 10 months
Kansas

Use calendars to record special daily events. They are convenient and can be used later to fill in baby books if desired.

Sue, RN, LCCE, and mother of Angie, age 20
Minnesota

Take a picture of your child EVERY month in the same place: next to a tree, sitting on a toy, next to a stuffed animal (my son was on a child's rocking chair). You will see a beautiful progression of your child's growth each month since your child will be sitting or standing next to something static size!

Amy, postnatal fitness instructor and mother of Aidan
Maryland

You can make your baby book even more special with a special congratulations note from the White House. This special note is free, and you can get it by simply sending your baby's name, address, and birth date to the following address:

White House Greetings Office
Room 39
Washington, DC 20500

Amy Clark, owner/founder of www.momadvice.com, and mother of Ethan, age 2
Indiana

I'm too busy for baby books, but I love collecting my children's voices on audio tapes. I have a little tape recorder, and I keep one tape per child on a shelf to grab when needed. I began recording their noises when I was pregnant with my first and could hear her heartbeat in utero at the doctor's office. I have her first cries from the day she was born, and now she's 7 years old and starting second grade. I interview her a few times a year, have her siblings talk and giggle, and now we've started taking the tape recorder along on family vacations so we all can share memories of our trips in the future. I treasure those tapes of my children's growing sounds, with their little giggles and voices from so long ago now…and someday I know these tapes will be a treasure for them, too.

Susan, homemaker, Web site manager, and mother of
Robin, age 7, Joshua, age 5, and Caleb, age 2
Oklahoma

I love to scrapbook my children's pictures. I write notes to them about every 6 months. I just write a page that shares what they like/dislike, some of their funny behaviors/words, etc. I also just tell them how much I love them and am enjoying every moment with them. I conclude the letter by writing a prayer for my child.

Stephanie, counselor LPC and mother of Jack, age 4, and Will, age 1½
Oklahoma

To get little ones to sit still and look darling for pictures, ask them to do a trick – something they're proud of doing, like clapping hands, saying how old they are, or making an animal sound. They'll be smiling and distracted long enough to take the picture, plus you can get sweet poses.

Alicia Bayer, writer, owner of www.magicalchildhood.com, and mother of Victoria, age 6, Annalee, age 4, and Jack, age 1
Minnesota

Don't just record major events and milestones and don't feel like everything has to go in the official "baby book." I keep a notebook on hand, and everytime my child does something — even little "somethings" like finding the bunnies on her PJ's — I jot it down with the date and my thoughts. As I put pictures in a scrapbook or catch up with the baby book, I'll be able to pull the info from my informal notebook.

Stacy, graphic artist, owner of Inkspot Creations, and mother of Julia, age 18 months
New Jersey

Write stories, dates, "firsts" down on a sticky note or slip of paper and store in one place until you can take the time to put them formally into a photo album or scrapbook. You'd be surprised how quickly you forget such details that you think you could never forget.

Heidi, courtesy of The Center for Conscious Parenting, www.cfcp.info, "run-outside-of-the-house" mom and mother of Heather, age 20 months
Oregon

Always have a camera on hand and write down important milestones. As your child grows, there will be countless times you will want to capture a perfect moment. Keep a camera (with film) nearby; otherwise, by the time you hunt it down, the moment will be lost. Likewise, keep a calendar on the refrigerator to record important moments as they happen. You may think you'll never forget that day your child first tasted prunes; but if you don't document it, trust me, you will forget. (I can barely remember what I need at the grocery store, much less when my child first waved bye-bye.) Write it down, write it down! You'll be glad you did.

Celeste Palermo, freelance writer and mother of Peyton, age 6, and Morgan, age 1
Colorado

Since I spend lots of time on the computer, I have started a folder in "Word" where I put in funny stories of things that my child has said or milestones she's accomplished, as well as sweet or memorable events that happen. Now, when I am sorting through pictures (digital or hard copy), I try to scrapbook them with a corresponding story. And if I don't get to my scrapbooking, at least I now have these stories for me to print out and put away for the future so I never forget all the little things I will always want to remember.

Christine, full-time diva and mother of Julia, age 2½, and Olivia, age 6 months
New Jersey

When the baby comes, jot down the first everything (hiccup, haircut, nail trim, smile, step, etc.). Keep a journal and write letters to the baby. This will be such a precious gift to your child someday!

Jill, full-time mother of Alison, age 1
Illinois

We made a video of our son every Sunday for the first year of his life. These "Sunday videos" captured everyday moments, family dinners, baths, and giggles. They also chronicled my son's amazing strength as he transformed on video from a 3-pound, 28-week preemie to a fragile 2-month-old baby, finally at home from the hospital with oxygen and lots of medical equipment; to the robust, chubby cheeked 6-month-old; to the mobile, strong 1-year-old. When we have another baby, we'll also take a picture every Sunday with the baby in the same location to really document change from week to week.

Connie, publisher and mother of Holden, age 3
New Jersey

In each child's bedroom, we marked the child's height, the date, and his/her age directly on the wall or on the molding. We did this several times throughout each year when our children were babies and then periodically throughout the years on birthdays or when anyone "felt" they were growing. The last measurement was taken on each child's last day of high school. When our first child was born, we lived in an apartment, and we actually took the whole piece of molding with us when we moved. We just nailed it to the new wall in the new house, and we still have it.

Angie, mother of 4 and grandmother of 2
Maine

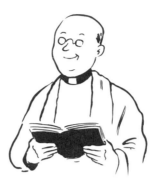

Spiritual Issues

In the myriad of parenting advice out there you will encounter many suggestions to approach your child in a way that seems unnatural or wrong to you. You'll hear things like "Let baby cry it out" or "Your baby is trying to manipulate you; show him who's boss." People will even cite Sacred Scripture to promote methods your heart tells you are abusive. Just remember that God has written His law on your heart and that's the law you need to follow. Your heart will tell you to hold and comfort your baby when she's upset, to nurse your baby whenever she asks to nurse, and, as she grows, to lovingly and gently guide her as she finds her way in life. That is God's voice within you. Listen to that voice. Listen to your heart.

Fernanda, mother of Laura, age 1
Colorado

For your baby's baptism, bris, baby naming, welcoming ceremony, or christening, in lieu of gifts, ask guests to bring a written wish, blessing, favorite poem, or quote for your child. Put the papers in a special box or container — we bought something that looks like a treasure box and decorated it —and read them to your child every year as part of a birthday ceremony or during transitional times when your child (or you) needs encouragement and strength.

Maryellen, senior art director and mother of
Matthew, age 20, and Kevin, age 19
Pennsylvania

The power of prayer is a very important force to introduce to young minds entering this ever changing world. Make sure that prayers (in whatever religion you may have in your home, even if the people raising the child are different cultures) are incorporated on a daily basis, either before bed or in the morning to start off their day. Do this activity with your child. This helps keep a positive attitude, helps reduce fear and anxiety, and instills the idea that there is a higher power to help us in our daily activities. So often we have a tendency as parents, and by no fault of our own, to make the child believe that we are their source in the universe. They need to know right away that this is not entirely so. So pick a short prayer for your children, blessing themselves and all other people and creatures; find an appropriate time of the day or night when the children are able to focus; and give your children the gift of letting them know that they can make a difference in this world.

**Cindy, educational assistant and mother of
Jaclyn, age 24, and Adam, age 21
New Jersey**

How to organize your own welcoming ceremony and still enjoy it? Take as long as you wish and you need to prepare, unless you have cultural traditions which indicate otherwise. Usually, there's no rush.

Allow yourself, as a new parent, to get over the initial sleepless nights and find your feet so you have energy and space in your day to prepare the ceremony. It is important to look forward to it.

Be bold and ask for help. Make it clear that if people are thinking about giving you or the baby a gift, what you would really appreciate is the gift of their time in the preparation of the ceremony. Maybe a friend could spend a couple of hours on the computer to type up and lay out beautifully your scribbled notes of what you plan to say on the day or the order of the ceremony with copies of poems and readings for people to take away. There may be some administration duties – sending out maps and travel directions, sending out lists of local B & B's – that friends could help with.

On the day, have a right-hand person whose job it is to keep everything ticking over and would get pleasure from doing that. This would save you headaches. This is the person who identifies car parking; who picks up the key to the community centre or hall and opens up for the caterers; or who remembers to switch the urn on so everything is ready when the guests arrive; and who, very possibly, gets volunteers to help clean up afterwards, deals with rubbish, makes any payments on your behalf, and takes the keys back!

Our book contains all the information you need to confidently go ahead and welcome a new life into the world: mythology of childbirth; baptism customs from the world's major faiths; ways to include children from other relationships in the ceremony; practical organization and stage management; numerous examples of how imaginative new parents have done it. Also included are ideas and inspiration on announcement cards, naming albums, your baby's time capsule, growing sticks, making papercuts and lanterns, using the seasons and the elements.

Here are some ideas for welcoming ceremonies for your baby.

The case for a spring/summer ceremony:

* You can have an "active" outdoor event.

* Friends attending can camp or bring a caravan to save costs.

* It's good for a family picnic, walk, or barbeque afterwards.

* It's easier to include elements of the earth, air, fire, and water.

* You can include flowers, flags, kites, and small boats.

* You will feel more relaxed taking your new baby out in good weather.

*Children can run around and let off steam with games, such as treasure hunts, as part of the day.

* Serve strawberry teas and homemade lemonade.

The case for an autumn/winter ceremony:

* This is a good time for those who prefer to gather in a hall or hotel for a tea party.

* The weather on the day will not affect the ceremony.

* You could bring your extended family together by renting a holiday house or cottage so the adults spend time together as well.

* It may be getting dark while you are celebrating the naming, so that suggests toffee apples, fireworks, lanterns, mulled wine, and storytelling.

* This is the best season for tree planting.

* Decorate using autumn berries, candles.

*You may get snow!

Sue Gill, co-editor of *The Dead Good Book of Namings and Baby Welcoming Ceremonies* and co-founder of Welfare State International, www.welfare-state.org and mother of two children and two grandchildren
United Kingdom

We were a bit unconventional. We waited until our daughters were each about 6 months old until we held the christenings. We had them both blessed at the church as soon as they were allowed in public areas, but we waited for the weather to change (warmer) to be able to have a nice "Welcoming" party for our babies with our family and friends.

Christine, full-time diva and mother of Julia, age 2½, and Olivia, age 6 months
New Jersey

Creating your own ceremonial space for a welcoming ceremony can give a powerful, natural focus for your ceremony. All that is required at a ceremony is our individual presence for the sharing of a special place and time. This quiet 'space' is at the heart of all ceremony. It's the point at which everything and everyone comes together in a magic way. It's the moment a child is named; the moment the toast has been proposed, and glasses travel towards lips. It's when the tears well, and we lose ourselves in that powerful mixture of joy and sadness. The trick is to extend, cultivate this moment, and that is the real ceremonial space: a combination of the physical, emotional, and spiritual. All the preparations and surroundings are a vessel built to launch it in. It's a magic dreamtime outside the busyness of everyday life in which affirmations can be made, changes and growth acknowledged, gateways passed through, and wounds healed. The simplest ceremonial space is instant. Stand in a circle and you have made the space. Bring nature inside. Use flowers and branches; weave twigs and greenery into garlands. Decorate a table as a focal point: use photographs, treasured family objects, and mementoes – reminders of what binds you together.

Sue Gill, co-editor of *The Dead Good Book of Namings and Baby Welcoming Ceremonies* and co-founder of Welfare State International, www.welfare-state.org and mother of two children and two grandchildren
United Kingdom

If you prefer your life without religion, select a humanist baby naming ceremony. A humanist baby naming ceremony is based on what we have in common – our humanity and human values. Each ceremony is a unique event: there is no set pattern or script, although the central part of the ceremony usually consists of a statement of commitment to the child's future by parents and supporting adults (the secular equivalent of godparents). Specially trained celebrants can write and then lead the ceremony, or you can create and lead it yourself. The British Humanist Association, based in the UK, in London, offers lots of helpful advice and has an excellent booklet entitled "New Arrivals," which gives lots of ideas and guidance. Parents who have chosen humanist ceremonies for their babies universally say that the experience was truly a good one, enabling them to hold a wonderful ceremony that allowed them to mark their baby's birth in a meaningful and sincere way according to their own beliefs and values.

Caroline, public relations consultant and aunt of nieces Emma, age 12, and Sarah, age 9, and nephews Rupert, age 16, and Kristopher, age 8
United Kingdom

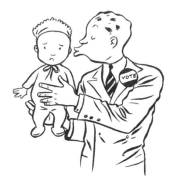

— Social Responsibility —

Now is the time to celebrate your new ferocious Mama grizzly bear-heart and act beyond the needs of your own child to the needs of all vulnerable children around the world. Though ensuring the health, education, and safety of all the world's children might sound like too big a job for some, with your expanded capacity, you're just the mom for the job. As you leave your insular world with your expanded awareness, it may be quite a shock to witness the discrepancy between how you are able to raise your child and the conditions under which some mothers of the world must try to nurture their children without access to healthcare, clean water, education, or safety. This is no time to waste even a second feeling guilty nor should guilt be your motivation. Let the solidarity of motherhood spur you to action. Look at this as a lifelong commitment of love, just as you have committed a lifetime of love to your own child. Getting involved is your best bet for ensuring peace and prosperity for your child and the world community of which your child is inextricably a part. Beyond that, your spirit is allowed to remain open and breathing when you do not shut out the cries of those less fortunate. Before I became consistently active, I often feared that I wouldn't be able to negotiate boundaries between my relatively abundant life and the unfathomable neediness of some of the world's population. That fear shriveled up and fell through the cracks when the greater focus of love shone down upon even my smallest actions. My fears only stayed large when I focused on them; once I changed my perspective, they appeared trivial in my peripheral vision. What dominated my vision was the excitement of possibilities, that I had the ability to actually bring about tangible change that would make the lives better for children and people I've never even met.

There are two ways to look at affecting change for those in need: first, through direct action and second, through advocating for systematic justice. Both approaches are worthwhile and essential in bringing about lasting change, but you might find one to be more your calling than the other. Try to match your talents, qualities, and appetite with the form of assistance that suits you best.

*Direct action includes efforts such as food banks, soup kitchens, women's shelters, and medical treatment facilities which offer immediate relief for suffering. The key with doing direct relief work is to integrate it into your new role as mother without compartmentalizing your volunteer work as necessarily separate. Be creative in discovering things you can do with your children. Indeed, the presence of your child may be the most healing thing you have to offer. My friend delivers lunches for Meals on Wheels, a program that offers nutritious meals to low-income seniors, with her children once a week, and it is the visit from her kids that these shut-in elderly recipients most value. For over two years now, my friend Juliana and I have led an art class once a month at a mental health outreach clubhouse, and we bring our children with us each time. In fact, it is the presence of the children that grants us all the permission to become childlike again in our artistic explorations. The obvious benefit of this, as well, is that you are engendering tolerance and compassion in your children. I have witnessed my son share his scissors so kindly with a mental health client during our art time, such that my mother heart was deeply touched. So put that baby in a backpack carrier and head for a soup kitchen. Visit a low-income nursing home with a group of your mother friends and sing nursery rhymes for your babies with the residents to the delight of all generations. Assist at a playgroup at a local women's shelter. Affect the world for the better and train the next generation of volunteers all in one simple act.

*Systematic Justice targets the systems of corporate and governmental policy that lead to the oppression that is often the root source of this suffering that direct assistance seeks to lessen. If working to improve the structure of government through which we shape policies and map out our nation's priorities is the thing that blows your skirt up, then you'll find ample opportunities to get involved. Just hop on-line at your own computer or at a computer at a local public library (the librarian can help you find these sites if you are unfamiliar navigating through the Web) and find out more about what you can do. Don't let intimidation slow you down; you don't have to be able to quote statistics to know what you value. You are smart enough right now to speak up for what you believe.

Here's some great contact information for you to get started! Phone numbers to memorize:

The White House (ask for the comment line): (202) 456-1414
Capitol Switchboard (to call your US legislators): (202) 224-3121
To find your elected officials, information on voting, and more:
www.vote-smart.org: everything you need to know to engage in the political process
www.verifiedvoting.org: working to make sure everyone's vote is counted
www.opensecrets.org: a nonpartisan account of who's funding whom
www.cdfactioncouncil.org/scorecard2003.pdf: a nonpartisan scorecard for members of Congress
www.grannyd.com: get involved in one of Granny D's voting projects
www.rockthevote.org: empowering young people to change their world

Federal government contacts:
www.whitehouse.gov: the President, VP, 1st Lady
www.senate.gov: US Senators
www.congress.gov: US Congress members
www.omb.gov: Office of Management and Budget (read your budget here)
www.childstats.gov: federal and state statistics and reports on children and their families
www.dod.gov: Department of Defense
www.epa.gov: Environmental Protection Agency
www.fda.gov: Food and Drug Administration
www.ed.gov: Department of Education
www.hhs.gov: Department of Health and Human Services

International bodies:
www.un.org: United Nations
www.icc-cpi.int: International Criminal Court

You may feel like a David poised against a Goliath, you may feel like your words fall upon a deaf world, you may fear that your cause will never triumph, but rest assured, "There is no chance of failing when one person raises their voice to bring dignity to another." These words were written by a mother, Stacy Carkonen, the night before she organized a Mothers Acting Up Mother's Day Parade to celebrate the rights of children. There is no winning or failing; there is just the evolution of becoming a fully compassionate member of the great human family. In that process it becomes quite clear, as members of the same family, that what is good for all is good for one. If that truth were to be unilaterally embraced, then the suffering caused by the selfishness of a few inflicted on the lives of many would cease to be. Until that time, let's keep our vision high, our hearts true, and our hands ready to reach out to another. Let us find our sustaining strength in the undeniable truth that it brings more oxygen to a mother's soul to work towards a better world for all children.

Beth Osnes, co-founder of Mothers Acting Up, part-time instructor of theatre at University of Colorado, and mother of Peter, age 11, Melisande, age 9, and Lerato, age 1, just adopted from South Africa!
Colorado

Important initiatives to share:

Millennium Goals (www.undp.org/mdg/) is an ambitious agenda for reducing poverty and improving lives that world leaders agreed on at the Millennium Summit in September 2000. For each goal, one or more targets have been set, most for 2015, using 1990 as a benchmark.

The Convention of the Rights of the Child (www.unicef.org/crc/crc.htm) is the most universally accepted human rights instrument in history. It has been ratified by every country in the world except two. (Guess who? ... The United States of America and Somolia)

What You Need to Know to Truly Leave No Child Behind (www.cdfactioncouncil.org/2003_ActionGuide.pdf) is an action guide complete with stats, actions and moving words from many. You won't regret printing the 60 pages!

All the facts you need to speak powerfully to everyone (including your father-in-law):

UNICEF Monitoring the Situation of Children and Women (www.childinfo.org) is the place to find all the info you need to assess the state of the world's children. Great charts, graphs, etc.

How Well Do Your Members of Congress Protect Children? (www.cdfactioncouncil.org/scorecard2003.pdf) is a nonpartisan scorecard for our members of Congress. This is the best place to find out if you are voting for a wolf in sheep's clothing!!

Beth Osnes, co-founder of Mothers Acting Up, part-time instructor of theatre at University of Colorado, and mother of Peter, age 11, Melisande, age 9, and Lerato, age 1, just adopted from South Africa!
Colorado

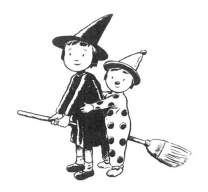

Beyond One

Be prepared. By this I mean: make a plan. The theme of my first round with motherhood was surprise: Surprise, the epidural's not working! Surprise, the breastfeeding's not working! Surprise, the working from home with a newborn isn't working! So for the next round, I tried to make those past surprises work for me by preparing myself better the second time. I made sure this time to not try to work from home four days after giving birth. I actually talked to my husband about how difficult it had been for me as a new mother the first time and even accepted his outlandish suggestion that he play a larger role in the crucial postpartum months after our second baby was born. I talked to a postpartum counselor before the baby came to make sure I had some objective support in place should things turn out to be surprising after all. I talked to my OB about all of these things so that we would be on the same page once the baby came, and I might be too chicken to admit I was overwhelmed. Having a plan in mind and being prepared helped me feel more in control, and it made the first few stressful weeks as a new mom of two that much more bearable.

Andrea J. Buchanan, author of *Mother Shock: Loving Every (Other) Minute of It* (Seal Press 2003), syndicated columnist, managing editor of LiteraryMama.com, and mother of two
Philadelphia

You think you can't possibly love another baby as much as you love your first one, but just try it…you'll see. You'll never BELIEVE how much love you have to give.

Tina, bookkeeper and mother of Fisher, age 5, Eli, age 2, and Sullivan, age 9 months
Texas

Don't be in a hurry to add to your family! I remember when my first was 18 months old, and she looked and acted so "grown up" that we decided we were ready to have our second. When our second was 18 months old, we realized that she was really still a baby and that having them 2½ years apart hadn't been such a great idea. I've heard parents say they want to get the early years "over with" and be done with diapers and breastfeeding, but babies don't want to get their babyhood "over with" since it's the only one they'll get. Instead of hurrying our babies – to be born at 40 weeks gestation, to sleep through the night (alone!), to eat solids, to learn to use the potty, to wean from the breast, to go to school, and on and on – try to enjoy these special little people. The time really does fly, and you can't get it back once it's gone. I look at pictures of our children and realize how precious and amazing they are at any age. Enjoy them and relax. It's the only time they're babies.

Kate, biologist and mother of Ursula, age 9, Sage, age 7, and Benno, age 3
Colorado

Notes to self when thinking about having another...

• Establish that healthy routine I keep meaning to implement — rest, exercise, inner calm BEFORE getting pregnant again— and actually go into pregnancy feeling confident and excited.

• Take time to process the idea that "I'm pregnant" and embrace it before sharing the good news with family and friends, which inevitably brings boat loads of unsolicited advice.

• Do something relaxing and rejuvenating every day.

• Embrace the changes and trust that my body knows what to do; after all, women have been having babies for centuries, and I have done this before.

• Resist the temptation to press on regardless. Listen to my body. When I'm tired, Rest!

• Surround myself with positive people support. DO NOT listen to the innumerable scary stories that others invariably feel compelled to share. Rehearse my response ahead of time!

• Plan AHEAD for postpartum care and enlist the help, support, and baby care wisdom from an experienced and warm hearted mother, friend, or doula like our friend Miss Karen. Tribal mothers get the help of all the other women in the tribe. We Americans are the only people crazy enough to try to do it all ourselves!

Linda, marketing communications and mother of
Braede Bailey, age 21 months
Connecticut

Special Deliveries

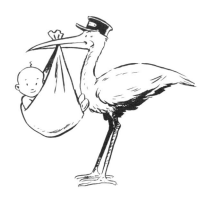

Adopting Baby

Be sure to use a certified adoption agency and not just an adoption attorney. With an agency you can attend classes that prepare you for the adoption process and for the handling of questions that will eventually arise after you have your child. You may not think that at the time you will use any of the advice or suggestions you are given, but then one day while explaining the process to a friend or stranger, all of a sudden you will be quoting something you read or something your caseworker told you.

Kristine, Pampered Chef consultant and mother of Isabel, age 2
Pennsylvania

Bringing Emil home from Romania at 21 months old was the best thing for our family. He was picked up at the airport with a teddy bear, and he still always has it in his room. Anyone considering adoption should do so. However, be prepared that these children may have special needs just like biological children may have special needs.

Elaine Emily Dreyfuss, speech pathologist and mother of Emil, age 7
New Jersey

Even when a child is adopted, the parents have instinct about this new baby's needs. Never give up finding just the right professional help who will work with you and your special knowledge of your baby.

Barb, mother of Jonas, age 25
Washington

I bathed with our adopted son, and then when we were ready for bed, we read together in our rocking chair every night. The bath gave us a physical bond, and the reading gave us an emotional bond. Reading is still an important way for us to spend our time – 5½ years later.

Alisa, mother of Benjamin, age 5½, and Lucas, age 2½
Texas

Bonding takes time. It's hard to hear that some people were "sure" immediately. Bonding happens over time. You and your baby need time to get to know one another and connect. It will happen.

Michelle, teacher and mother of Tyler, age 17 months, born at 30 weeks
and met by his adopted parents at 2 days old
California

Don't be afraid to use the word "adoption" around your child, family, and friends. Include everyone in the process. We don't tell our daughter everyday that she is adopted, but when a friend adopts a child, we see something on TV, or on the anniversary of the day we brought her home, we say, "We are so happy we adopted you. You have brought so much joy into our lives, and we are so proud to have been chosen to be your parents." If you whisper the word, your child will pick up on it. Tell your child her story. We all have one.

Kristine, Pampered Chef consultant and mother of Isabel, age 2
Pennsylvania

My sister-in-law asked me, "What was the most surprising thing about becoming a mother?" I thought for only a second, and the answer was so quick. We had waited so long for a child, and the adoption process took longer than we wanted as well. Perhaps my sister-in-law was fishing for the sleeplessness or the sense that very little gets accomplished in a day besides feeding, cleaning, and more of the same. Yet for me, clearly the most surprising thing was that I didn't need to give birth to feel this connected to my precious little girl! She is so much a part of me that I sometimes forget that we never shared the same bodily space! You can never quite explain this to a couple struggling with infertility. It is only in the experience of becoming a mother through adoption that you may find this joy as well.

Melissa, interfaith minister and mother of Annamika, age 5
Pennsylvania

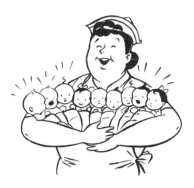

Expecting Multiples

Relax! Breathe! My twins are now eight months old; and even though they are here and having them has been easier than I expected, I can still easily recall the shock and amazement I felt when I was given the news at 10 weeks that there was more than one baby in there! I started reading everything that I could on twin pregnancy, delivery, and beyond. Twin pregnancies are often thought to be very risky by medical professionals, but I felt it was really important for me to stay in tune with my body and listen to myself just as much as I listened to the professionals. Although I made sure to do everything I needed to do to ensure the health and safety of my babies, I also made sure that I asked a lot of questions and ultimately made my own decisions regarding my care.

Kathy, mother of Alejandro, age almost 3, and twins Nieves and Paloma, age 9 months
New Jersey

When you find out that you are pregnant with twins (or more), take a tour of the Neonatal Intensive Care Unit (NICU) at your hospital and ask detailed questions about procedures since you have more of a likelihood of having children spend time in the NICU. It made a huge difference to me to not be scared with all the other overwhelming things I was going through the day my twins were born to know that the NICU was a warm and welcoming place for my daughter to go instead of the cold, sterile place I had imagined.

Tara, mother of twins Caroline and Ryan, age 2½
Washington

When I found out I was having twins again I just laughed! My best advice for mothers of multiples is sleep when they sleep and don't panic… we have two hands for a reason! Sometimes I wish I was an octopus!

**Jennifer, stay-at-home mother of
twins Karlie and Brooke, age 4, and twins Morgan and Emily, age 1
Georgia**

Surprise! There's two babies! Do research for your nearest Mothers of Multiples Club! These women are there to offer support and encouragement! Just knowing that your experiences are all quite "normal" makes everything so much easier.

**Dawn, domestic engineer and mother of
Miranda, age 11, Vinnie, age 7, and Alicia and Chad, age 4
Ohio**

Good nutrition (along with rest) is absolutely the best thing, in my opinion, that you can do for yourself and your babies while you're pregnant. Certainly, I'm all for giving in to cravings — I mean, I am the same woman who ate a whole ham in one sitting while pregnant with my son — but by setting an overall foundation of good nutrition, you're giving your baby the very best from the get-go. I found with my second pregnancy — twins — that eating a high amount of protein was essential. High consumption of protein should NOT be mistaken for any kind of carb-counting diet. Rather, I was following the Brewer pregnancy diet. After finding information on the Brewer diet online, I called their "hotline" and had a lovely conversation with Dr. Brewer himself, who has been an OB/GYN for over 50 years. His diet is tailored for a single pregnancy, but he was happy to fine-tune it for the special needs of my pregnancy: In addition to having twins, we had a condition called Twin to Twin Transfusion Syndrome, which may be controlled (some experts believe) largely through nutrition before more invasive procedures are required. The protein helped keep my energy levels up, kept my legs from cramping, and provided the building blocks for creating my two beautiful babies. If you're uncomfortable with what you're eating or are simply unsure if it's adequate, ask your midwife or doctor for a referral to a registered dietician or dietetic technician. These specialists have the tools available to them to help analyze your diet, and they will be able to give suggestions and work with you to provide optimal nutrition throughout your pregnancy.

**Kathleen, mother of Alejandro, age almost 3,
and twins Nieves and Paloma, age 9 months
New Jersey**

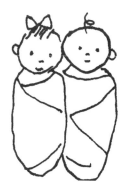

Care of Multiples

Knowing you'll have two babies to care for, maternity ward nurses are extra supportive and generous. We got lots of Vaseline tubes, alcohol swabs, snot-sucking syringes, formula samples, Lasinoh (nipple ointment for nursing moms), disposable changing pads, sterilized gauze pads for our son's circumcision maintenance – the list goes on and on. Don't be embarrassed to ask!

Cheryl Lage, Web host of www.twinsights.com, a site for new and expecting twin moms, and full-time mother of fraternal twins, Darren and Sarah Jane, age 3
Virginia

Screen your phone calls. People will understand that with infant twins, you are juggling. Return calls when you are rested, at a convenient point, and can carry on a decent conversation. No one knows your schedule, but they do care, and they want you to know it. Consider e-mail updates. You may have a great window of opportunity and be wide awake at 4:00 am. They'll get a kick out of the fact that you want them "in the loop" and that you composed the correspondence at such a crazy hour.

Cheryl Lage, Web host of www.twinsights.com, a site for new and expecting twin moms, and full-time mother of fraternal twins, Darren and Sarah Jane, age 3
Virginia

When the babies are first brought home from the hospital, let them sleep in one crib for the first few months – they will sleep better. After all, they have been sleeping together for the first nine months!

Stephanie, full-time mother of twins Edward and Harold, age 6
Massachusetts

With twins, you need your sleep. There is no "passing off to Dad" when there are two babies in the house. Our pediatrician suggested the following for our 6-week-old twin boys; and after just a few weeks, our twin boys were sleeping through the night. Always put them to sleep awake. They need to know that their crib is where they should fall asleep. Let them cry, but only if you know there is nothing wrong (they are not sick, they have a clean diaper, etc.). After 20 minutes of crying, enter the room and rub their bellies, speaking softly and soothing them until they stop. Leave the room and repeat as needed. Only enter the room every 20 minutes. Warning: it will break your heart! The first couple of nights we repeated this pattern for 2½ hours. Then after the third night, for one hour; and after six nights, they were sleeping 7 am to 7 pm and getting up once at 3 am for a feed! At exactly (to the day!) 3 months corrected age, they slept 7 am to 7 pm without waking up. They are now 6 months old (4 months corrected) and often sleep for 14 hours per night!

Heidi, human resources professional and mother of twins
Keegan John and Kade Peter, age 6 months
Canada

When my twin boys were about 3 weeks old, we found out real quick that putting them on the same schedule worked wonderfully! We bottle fed and used their car seats for nighttime feedings. We sat in the middle and fed both at the same time. We would put one in the swing after eating while his brother was getting his diaper changed, and he would stay there until it was his turn for a change. To this day they are still very patient waiting their turn.

Janet, homemaker and mother of identical twins Tyler and Taylor, age 8
Georgia

If you have identical twin or multiple infants or toddlers, it is completely acceptable to dress them alike…they will not know the difference, and you should enjoy their "twinship."

Debbie and Lisa Ganz, twin experts
New York

I am a mother of four children. The last children I had are identical twin girls. I learned a lot after my first two. I was losing lots of sleep and not getting any rest with them. I read books and found an article about how to get your baby to sleep all night. It was a great one, and it paid off big time. It said never put your baby in the bed with you. Your baby will get used to being in the bed with parents, and it will be extremely hard to get him/her to sleep in his/her own bed when the time comes. Another point was always feed your baby and change his/her diaper before bedtime, make sure the baby is going to be okay, and always put your baby on his/her back, never face down. Leave the room and check on baby throughout the night. I used a baby monitor beside my bed so if I heard something, I would check on my baby. If one of my twins cried, I would go ahead and feed her and change her diaper. I would then wake the other twin up and feed her. Actually, I fed them at the same time. I did this for about two weeks, and they were sleeping all night at 2½ months. I was blessed with two good twins, and I got my rest, and it was wonderful.

Beverly, mother of twins Brittany and Tiffany, age 4
Virginia

As a mother of identical twins, I hate to admit it, but I have mixed up their names. In certain situations this is very dangerous. For instance, if one of your twins is running toward the street and you call out the wrong name, he/she may not respond. So here is some great advice that someone gave to me. Put them in different color shoes or use different color shoelaces. That way if you need to get their attention in an emergency situation, you will know immediately whose name to call out. Even if you don't dress them alike, shoes are a constant article of clothing that is easily identifiable. Other advice that I have gotten about this is to dress each one in the same color all the time – one twin in red and green, one in yellow and blue. However, I find that my boys like to pick out their own clothes and are very opinionated on the colors they choose to wear, so that hasn't worked out for us.

Jennifer, graphic artist and mother of twins Kyle and Parker, age 3
Kentucky

Always feed twin babies at the same time. If one wakes, then wake and feed the other one, too, even if the other baby is sound asleep. Keep them on the same schedule.

Shannon, stay-at-home mother of Virginia, age 5, Davis, age 3,
and twins Catherine and Jack, age 3 months
Georgia

As the mother of twin girls, I absolutely hated cleaning the high chairs and booster seats after every meal. As soon as my girls were old enough to sit without being strapped in, I ordered each of them one of the booster seats used in many restaurants. It is called a dual booster seat. It is the two-sided seat the offers a choice in heights so that they could sit at the dining table or flip it over and sit at the breakfast bar. Better yet, it is a one-piece molded unit that can be easily washed in the kitchen sink. It comes in many colors, including the basic beige that will go with any décor. You can order one from most restaurant supply stores. What a joy not to have to unstrap those ugly primary-colored seats anymore and get all the mess out from under them and out of every little crevice!

Debbie, full-time mother of twins Laura and Natalie, age 3
Alabama

I know it may sound mean, but it's the only way you'll get any sleep. When one child wakes in the night, feed, change, and then back to bed the first one goes. Then you wake the other child: change, feed, and then back to bed that one goes, too! Otherwise, you could be getting up all night long. It worked for me.

Tina, account manager and mother of twins Rachel and Anastasia, age 14
New York

Sleep when the babies sleep. Forget about your grown-up ritual of only sleeping when it is dark outside. Nighttime interruptions in the first few months with newborn twins will be lengthy and frequent. Learn to at least rest when they do, regardless of the time on the clock.

Cheryl Lage, Web host of www.twinsights.com, a site for new and expecting twin moms, and full-time mother of fraternal twins, Darren and Sarah Jane, age 3
Virginia

Take a "V" cushion and place it across your lap with each side of the cushion resting on either side of you. Place one baby on one side with his/her head near the "V" and feet going behind you and the other baby in the same position on the other side. This way you can breastfeed two babies at the same time and have more time for yourself in between feeds.

Natasha, driving instructor and mother of identical twins, Sadie and Ruby, age 4
Hertfordshire, England

After sleepily feeding one baby twice while the other missed a feeding and changing twice, we realized we needed to make (and use!) a simple chart. No matter what time we fed or changed a baby, especially at 4 am, we just put the time and a check mark by their name. Everyone stayed dry, fed, and happy.

Victoria, mother of twins Jane and Susanne, age 5½
California

Definitely plan on going out with your babies and do so often. Just be sure to allow yourself abundant time—not only for getting yourself and two babies in and out of the car on both ends of your trip, but for onlookers and well-wishers to ogle your twins and offer their congratulations throughout. With two infants in tow, they will, believe me! Don't ever plan on squeezing too many errands into a narrow window of time. Err on the side of making numerous small trips. Try to revel in, rather than be inconvenienced by, the well-meaning attention of strangers while out and about with your babies. A cheerful, relaxed, socially-at-ease twin mommy often results in cheerful, relaxed, socially-at-ease twins. (Be warned: The reverse is also true!)

Cheryl Lage, Web host of www.twinsights.com, a site for new and expecting twin moms, and full-time mother of fraternal twins, Darren and Sarah Jane, age 3
Virginia

Find a support group for Mothers/Parents of Multiples. The wealth of information and support along with the friendships formed by both parents and children is incredible.

Marcy, mother of Brittany, age 7, Thomas, age 7, and Megan, age 19 months
New York

Parents of multiples will face particular problems with raising siblings of the same age which will require coping abilities different from those with single children. However, once parents are used to the idea of two or more babies instead of one, they feel it's not really "Double Trouble" or "Triple Trouble," but "Twice as Nice" or "Triple the Fun."

Jennifer Noonan, director of publications for the Australian Multiple Birth Association (AMBA)
Australia

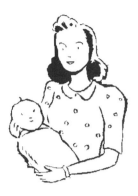

Single Parenting

Plan your budget based on your income, not your child support. The child support you receive can be used for extras and emergencies, just in case the father or non-custodial parent decides to stop paying.

Robbie, mother of Holl, age 2
Texas

As a single mom, I had to work and needed my own sleep to do that. What really helped me was something I learned from Penelope Leach in her book *Your Baby and Child*. If my baby started crying in the middle of the night, I would go in and determine if he was okay. Then I would comfort him with a few soothing words and a rub on the back. Then I would leave, set the timer for 15 minutes and fall back asleep. If he was still crying when the timer went off, I would go back and do the same thing again. He soon learned that mom was nearby and would comfort him, but wouldn't take him out of bed. This helped me feel like I was responding to his need for comfort without disrupting my whole night. It was essential to our successfully navigating those early months.

Lynne, social work administrator and mother of Brint, age 18
Alabama

Find a single mommy support group. They will understand what you're going through a lot better than your married or co-habitating friends.

Robbie, mother of Holl, age 2
Texas

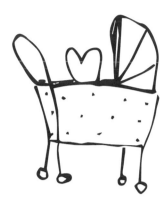

Special Needs Baby

Remember to take care of yourself. As the mother of a special needs child, you need to remember to take care of yourself as well. Always make time for at least an hour a week of downtime. It may be as simple as a long, warm, soothing bath or a manicure. I found that raising a special needs child requires as much mental work as physical, and my time down was my sanity.

Wyndella, mother of Brianna
Delaware

When you are expecting a baby, we often take for granted that our child will be typical, so it can come as quite the shock when you are told that your child has special needs. This happened to us when we found out our child has Down Syndrome. Being that my husband and I are still in our twenties, the possibility had never even crossed our minds. One thing to remember, though, is that no matter what, this is YOUR child, and you will love him or her with all your heart. Another thing to note is that having a child can help you tap into your own sense of compassion and understanding the way nothing else could. And finally, having a child with special needs is a true blessing...you will experience unconditional love and celebrate every milestone in a way you never knew was possible.

Katrina, graphic designer and mother of Kristina, age 3, and Brant, age 1
Canada

Finding out that a child has been born with a disability or that a previously healthy child has suffered an injury or disease that causes a disability can be the most traumatic moment in a parent's life. Shock is usually the first thing people experience. After coming to grips with the shock of their situation, many parents come to feel that their expectations have been dashed, that they are failures as parents, or that their family has been destroyed. Uncertainty, blame, or jealousy may arise. These emotions, however, are a normal part of a "mourning" process that many parents of children with disabilities go through. If you have these feelings, remember that you are not the only ones who feel this way, and that you will get over them. You can adjust more quickly by obtaining accurate information, sharing your feelings openly with others, seeking professional counseling, and, most importantly, having open discussions with all members of your immediate family. It is not the end of the world, and many families have become stronger, more loving, and more closely knit because of a disability in the family. The disability gave them the opportunity to work together to help out their loved one, and the entire family shared in the gains that are made by the child. The most important factor in a family's success is the motivation to succeed. If a child realizes that his parents always encourage success and will not be satisfied with anything less than his best effort, he will be motivated to succeed. Never settling for failure becomes part of his character, and his self-esteem will be enhanced and maintained.

Dr. Mark Nagler, Ph.D., disabilities expert and father
Ontario, Canada

"Special Needs" does not mean that life is over. If by chance your child is born with a special need, say, Rett Syndrome or some other curve ball in the genetic ballgame of life, take some time to grieve the image of what you lost and reflect on what a gem you've got. Then embrace your child and get ready for an amazing ride. LIFE IS FAR FROM OVER, but a new reality has just begun.

Courtney, certified birth doula and mother of
Blythe, age 2½ and born with Rett Syndrome,
and Fiona, age 1 and born with Spunky Little Girl Syndrome
Texas

Send us your tips!

Be a part of new books in the MOTHERS KNOW BEST series.

We are seeking tips on:
toddlers and preschoolers
adoption
school-age children
multiples
and
special needs children

We can also accept tips from dads on all aspects of parenting and surviving your partner's pregnancy.

Please fill out this submission form or submit tips via our Web page at http://www.mothersknowbest.net. We encourage you to copy this sheet as needed for additional tips or to pass on to other wise mothers so they can share their tips. We can accept three tips per person. If your tip worked for your child at a certain age, please list that age.

If you do NOT want your last name listed, please do not include it on your submission. State or country information must be included. Also, please make sure you provide some way to reach you — phone or e-mail — so we can contact you if we have a question about your submission. Your contact information WILL NOT be shared with anyone.

Please mail sheet to:

Small Potatoes Press
401 Collings Avenue
Collingswood, NJ 08108

You may also fax your tips to 856-869-5247 or submit them via our Web site www.mothersknowbest.net.

Questions?
Call us at 856-869-5207 or e-mail to
info@smallpotatoespress.com.

Visit our Web site at www.mothersknowbest.net.

Subject _____

Tip _____

_____

_____

_____

_____

_____

_____

_____

Name _____

*Profession _____

Web site _____

*Address _____

*City _____

State _____ *Zip _____ Country _____

E-mail _____

Phone _____

*Child/Children's First Name(s) and Age(s) _____

_____

_____

_____

I agree to have the above tips and my name and child/children's first name(s)
and age(s) printed in the proposed book as well as future publications and
promotions. I understand that there will be no financial renumeration or
compensation for such inclusion, and I will seek none. I will not hold the publisher
liable for any errors or typographical mistakes. Small Potatoes Press has the right
to restrict the inclusion of any tip.

Signed _____ Date _____

*optional

About the Authors

A graduate of Johnson & Wales University, Connie Correia Fisher is the coauthor of five cookbooks and served as editor and designer of the award-winning cookbook *Joe Brown's Melange Cafe Cookbook*. She is the founding publisher/editor of *Cuizine* magazine. Connie is a lazy scrapbook wannabe and lives in Collingswood, New Jersey, with her husband and amazing toddler son.

Joanne Correia is Connie's mom and the former executive editor of *Cuizine* magazine. She and Connie are the authors of five cookbooks. Joanne is a full-time employee of the Cherry Hill Board of Education, has just taken up jogging, has four kids and four grandchildren, and — according to her daughter — is the best mommy in the world. Joanne lives in Cherry Hill, New Jersey, with her husband.